THE HEALTHCARE EXECUTIVE'S GUIDE TO ACO STRATEGY

COKER GROUP

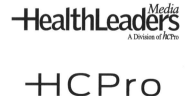

Coker Group, Author

Carrie Vaughan, Editor

Bob Wertz, Managing Editor

Matt Cann, Group Publisher

Doug Ponte, Cover Designer

Mike Mirabello, Graphic Artist

Matt Sharpe, Production Manager

Shane Katz, Art Director

Jean St. Pierre, Senior Director of Operations

Advice given is general. Readers should consult professional counsel for specific legal, ethical, or clinical questions. Arrangements can be made for quantity discounts. For more information, contact:

HCPro, Inc.

75 Sylvan Street, Suite A-101

Danvers, MA 01923

Telephone: 800/650-6787 or 781/639-1872

Fax: 800/639-8511

E-mail: *customerservice@hcpro.com*

HCPro, Inc., is the parent company of HealthLeaders Media.

Visit HealthLeaders Media online at *www.healthleadersmedia.com*

03/2012
21964

Contents

Contents

Contents

About the Authors

Max Reiboldt, CPA

Max Reiboldt provides sound financial and strategic solutions to hospitals, medical practices, health systems, and other healthcare entities through keen analysis and problem solving. Working with organizations of all sizes, Reiboldt engages in consulting projects with organizations nationwide. His expertise encompasses employee and physician employment and compensation, physician-hospital affiliation initiatives, business and strategic planning, mergers and acquisitions, practice operational assessments, ancillary services development, physician-hospital organization, independent practice association and management services organization development, practice appraisals, and negotiations for acquisitions and sales. He also performs financial analyses for healthcare entities as well as buy/sell agreements and planning arrangements for medical practices.

Reiboldt is president and CEO of Coker Group and has led the firm's growth since the late 1990s to its position today as one of the leading healthcare consulting firms in the United States and abroad. He is a prolific author and accomplished public speaker on healthcare management topics.

Reiboldt has authored or contributed to many of Coker Group's 50-plus books. Recent titles include *Financial Management of the Medical Practice*, Third Edition (© 2011, AMA Press); *Reimbursement Management: Improving the*

Success and Profitability of Your Practice (© 2011, AMA Press); *RVUs at Work: Relative Value Units in the Medical Practice* (© 2010, Greenbranch Publishing); and *Physician Entrepreneurs: Strength in Numbers–Consolidation and Collaboration Strategies to Grow Your Practice* (© 2008, HealthLeaders Media).

A graduate of Harding University, Reiboldt is a licensed certified public accountant (CPA) in Georgia and Louisiana and a member of the American Institute of Certified Public Accountants, Healthcare Financial Management Association, and American Society of Appraisers.

Sue Hertlein

Sue Hertlein is a manager at Coker Group, and she works with physicians and hospitals across the country on numerous technology, strategic planning, and assessment projects. Hertlein's experience includes operational and workflow analysis, practice management and electronic health record (EHR) assessments, and readiness evaluations, vendor analysis/recommendation, vendor contact negotiations, systems testing, implementation, project management, and community needs assessments. In addition to her client work, Hertlein also manages Coker's research and assists in obtaining information on new situations that affect the healthcare industry, such as healthcare reform, meaningful use/EHR incentives, accountable care organizations (ACO), and physician-hospital alignment.

Hertlein has been a contributing author to several of Coker Group's 50-plus books. Recent titles include: *The Complete EMR Selection Guide* (© 2011 HIMSS); *Financial Management of the Medical Practice*, Third Edition (© 2011,

AMA Press); *Starting, Buying, and Owning the Medical Practice* (© 2012, AMA Press). Hertlein has also authored numerous published articles and white papers. She has also been a featured speaker on subjects such as EHRs, healthcare automation, ACOs, return on investment for EHRs, and employee-based topics, such as improving productivity, employee embezzlement, and staff training.

Contributors

Justin Chamblee, MAcc, CPA, senior manager

Justin Chamblee works with clients in a variety of strategic and financial areas, mainly dealing with physician compensation and hospital-physician transactions. He holds a Bachelor of Business Administration degree in accounting and a Master of Accounting from Abilene Christian University. He is licensed as a CPA in the state of Texas and is a member of the American Institute of Certified Public Accountants.

Jeffrey Daigrepont, senior vice president

Jeffery Daigrepont specializes in healthcare automation, strategic planning, operations, and deployment of fully integrated information systems for medical practices and hospitals. For fiscal year 2009, he chaired the ambulatory information steering committee (AISC) of the Healthcare Information and Management Systems Society (HIMSS). In addition, as the ambulatory committee liaison for fiscal year 2009 to the Annual Conference Education Committee, he represented the HIMSS ambulatory and AISC members.

Aimee Greeter, MPH, manager

As an integral part of Coker's financial services service line, Aimee Greeter works on a variety of consulting projects, including financial consulting, hospital accounts, and practice management initiatives, as well as research and writing for various client projects. She holds a Master of Public Health in health policy and management from the Rollins School of Public Health at Emory University. She is an honors graduate of Michigan State University, where she attained a Bachelor of Science in human biology.

Craig Hunter, senior vice president

Craig Hunter serves as Coker's business development leader, and he works with health systems, hospital-based networks, multi- and single-specialty groups, and independent physician practices facilitating phases of integration and practice development, including mergers, strategic planning, management reviews, and negotiations. He speaks frequently to health system and physician executives, administrators, and other healthcare personnel, and is a published author on practice management topics such as compensation, integration, and physician recruitment and employment.

Greg Mertz, FACMPE

Greg Mertz has more than 30 years of healthcare industry experience. His expertise is in performance improvement of complex physician organizations in both hospital-affiliated and private settings. He has also advised clients on the business impact of industry trends, the beneficial impact of technology adoption, and the various models available for physician compensation. Mertz holds bachelor degrees in business and psychology from Gettysburg College, a Master of Business Administration/HMSA from Widener University, and is a member of the Medical Group Management Association.

Mark Reiboldt, MSc, senior vice president

Mark Reiboldt works in Coker's financial services group where he advises healthcare facilities through the transaction process, including due diligence, valuation and fairness opinion, as well as general strategic financial advisory. He received a Bachelor of Arts in political science from Georgia State University and a Master of Science in financial economics from the University of London. He is a Financial Industry Regulatory Authority–registered securities dealer with Series 7, 63, 65, and 79 licenses.

About Coker Group

Coker Group, a national healthcare consulting firm, helps providers achieve improved financial and operational results through sound business principles (*www.cokergroup.com*). Coker's team members are proficient, trustworthy professionals with expertise and strengths in various areas, including healthcare, technology, finance, and business knowledge. Coker represents three service lines: Coker Consulting, Coker Capital Advisors, and Coker Technology. Through these service areas, Coker consultants enable providers to concentrate on patient care.

Service areas include, but are not limited to: hospital-physician alignment, ACO readiness, capital advisory, strategic financial advisory and analysis, practice management, mergers/acquisitions and due diligence, compensation, pre- and post-merger integration, strategic IT planning and review, vendor vetting, managed IT services, hospital operations, medical staff development and executive search.

Coker Group's nationwide client base includes major health systems, hospitals, physician and specialty groups, and solo practitioners in a full spectrum of engagements. Coker has gained a reputation since 1987 for thorough, efficient, and cost-conscious work to benefit its clients both financially and operationally. The members of the firm pride themselves on their client profile of recognized and respected healthcare professionals throughout the industry. Coker Group is dedicated to helping healthcare providers face today's challenges for tomorrow's successes.

Acknowledgments

Books written by employees of Coker Group are always touched by the many people both inside and outside our organization. This work is no exception. First, we would like to give special thanks to the contributions made by our fellow Coker family members for their dedication to researching the content offered in this publication: Justin Chamblee, Jeffery Daigrepont, Aimee Greeter, Craig Hunter, Greg Mertz, and Mark Reiboldt. In addition to our primary authors, Max Reiboldt and Sue Hertlein, we thank these contributors for extending their knowledge from their many years of work in medical practices and physician networks.

Kay Stanley, who has contributed to Coker's 50-plus books since Coker's publishing initiative began in the early 1990s, has served as editor and project manager. Sue Hertlein spent hours researching the accountable care organization proposed regulations to ensure that readers have the most up-to-date information. Trish Hutcherson ably managed the team of contributors.

Special thanks and recognition goes to key players in the Norton Healthcare and Dartmouth-Hitchcock organizations, including Kevin Stone, director of accountable care development, Dartmouth-Hitchcock; George Y. Hersch, system vice president, material management, Norton Healthcare; Ben Yandell, PhD, CQE, vice president, material management, Norton Healthcare; and Ken Wilson, MD,

Acknowledgments

system vice president, clinical effectiveness and quality, Norton Healthcare. Their input and willingness to share information proved invaluable.

Finally, we appreciate the confidence placed in Coker Group by HealthLeaders Media to relay accurate and pertinent market information.

Preface

With the passing of the Patient Protection and Affordable Care Act (PPACA), signed into law by President Barack Obama in 2010, the healthcare industry has been in preparation mode for the changes that will ensue as the law goes into effect. One of the principles of the Act is the concept of accountable care and, more specifically, the establishment of accountable care organizations (ACO) for Medicare beneficiaries under the fee-for-service program. Although ACOs take up only seven pages of the massive new health law, they have become one of the most talked-about provisions.

This latest model for delivering services offers physicians and hospitals financial incentives to provide good quality care to Medicare beneficiaries while keeping down costs. ACOs would make providers jointly accountable for the health of their patients, giving them strong incentives to cooperate and save money by avoiding unnecessary tests and procedures. For ACOs to work, they have to seamlessly share information. Those that save money while also meeting quality targets would keep a portion of the savings. But some providers could also be at risk of losing money under Track 2 of the Centers for Medicare & Medicaid Services (CMS) program.

In March 2011, the CMS released its proposed guidelines, which provided a draft of what an ACO would look like. This was an exploratory time used to iron out some of the details. Late in 2011, CMS released the final rule for Medicare ACOs; however, some items are not fully finalized. (**Note:** CMS is still finalizing some items that will be released at a later date, and CMS and the Office of Inspector General [OIG] have released an "interim final rule with comment period" [60 days] regarding anti-kickback laws and some suggested waivers.)

With the CMS ACO initiative scheduled to launch in April 1, 2012 (followed by the second wave of ACO entities on July 1, 2012), the formation of ACOs has already begun. Hospitals, physician practices, and insurers across the country are announcing their plans to form private ACOs. Many healthcare providers have formed these private ACOs prior to the release of even the proposed CMS regulations so they could be one of the first groups to move forward with this new, innovative model in patient care. They believe that being patient-centered, improving the quality of care, working in tandem with their peers (and competitors in some cases), and reducing costs are the right things to do. Some of them also chose the private model to avoid more in-depth government regulations. Other providers are taking a wait-and-see perspective to evaluate the success (or failure) of the private ACOs and also to gain a further understanding of the financial implications of forming and/or joining a CMS ACO entity. There is no doubt that this new generation of healthcare models is under careful review from all types of providers because there are many questions to be answered and results to analyze.

The purpose of this book is to focus on what we know about ACOs at this early stage. The subject matter addresses ACOs in general and discusses various aspects of private and CMS entities. With the release of the final regulations in late 2011, there is a greater emphasis on the CMS Shared Savings Program.

Accountable Care Organization—An Overview

The concept of accountable care organizations (ACO) is gaining a great deal of attention in the reshaping of American health policy. Although this term is becoming common in healthcare delivery system vernacular, it remains an unknown concept to the vast majority of the public, including many physicians. The ACO label was invented late in 2006 during a discussion at a public meeting of the Medicare Payment Advisory Commission. Included in the Patient Protection and Affordable Care Act (PPACA), this concept has become the most talked-about new reimbursement and healthcare delivery system paradigm in some time.

Although ACOs may seem new, many of the concepts and basic tenets have been around since the beginning of the HMO movement in the 1970s. The primary difference between HMOs and ACOs, at least for the foreseeable future, will be their size. Whereas HMOs generally have enrollees in the hundreds of thousands, the ACO has so far been defined as having a much smaller number of enrollees, with a minimum of 5,000. We will sort out the new packaging and provide the reader with a clear path to understanding the new dynamic.

What Is an ACO?

Multiple definitions of ACOs seem to be appearing, but most have basic premises in common. An ACO by definition is an integrated healthcare delivery system (sound familiar?) that contracts to provide a full continuum of services to a defined patient population with specific reimbursement (financial) incentives established for meeting both quality and expense/cost targets.

ACOs are quickly emerging as the future care delivery and economic-reimbursement model to address the stressful challenges of increasing healthcare costs and a disparate and fragmented healthcare delivery system. As a result, healthcare providers will face new challenges and pending requirements, which call for more provider consolidation in order to demonstrate cost containment and high-quality patient care. ACOs will assume responsibility for both costs and quality as they provide care to a defined population. ACO provisions were included in the PPACA, which was signed into law March 2010. Under the title "Shared savings program," CMS is authorized to create an ACO "program" by no later than January 1, 2012. Under voluntary demonstration projects, the qualifying ACOs will be eligible for additional reimbursement as a result of a percentage of savings they realize through attainment of certain quality and savings thresholds. PPACA also established the CMS Center for Innovation, which is anticipated to provide funding for other projects with variable financing models, including bundled payments and a form of reimbursement prevalent in the 1980s and '90s: capitation.

The proposed CMS regulations were issued on March 31, 2011, followed by a comment period, with the final regulations issued on October 20, 2011. CMS reviewed each comment submitted and was influenced by many of the responders. As a result, CMS made some positive changes to the regulations with the hope that they would entice more providers to participate in the ACO program.

The Logic of ACOs

ACOs are a response to trends in the cost of healthcare, which has risen every year since 1989, as Figure 1.1 illustrates. This trend is one of the major drivers of both

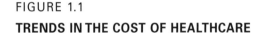

FIGURE 1.1

TRENDS IN THE COST OF HEALTHCARE

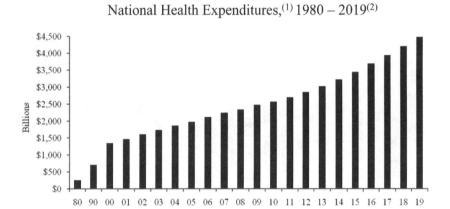

National Health Expenditures,[1] 1980 – 2019[2]

Source: Available at www.aha.org/aha/research-and-trends/chartbook/ch1.html. *Accessed January 13, 2011.*

[1] *Years 2009–2019 are projections.*
[2] *CMS completed a benchmark revision in 2006, introducing changes in methods, definitions, and source data that are applied to the entire time series (back to 1960). For more information on this revision, see* www.cms.hhs.gov/NationalHealthExpendData/downloads/benchmark.pdf

American Hospital Association, TrendWatch Chartbook 2010, Trends in the Overall Health Care Market, Chart 1.8. www.aha.org/aha/research-and-trends/chartbook/ch1.html. *Accessed January 13, 2011.*

government and private insurers as they seek ways, through the reimbursement system, to address increasing costs. We could adjust to rising costs for a certain period of time; however, we can no longer continue to tolerate and accept such increases. Many experts say we are at the end of our proverbial rope.

Recognizing that the number of Medicare enrollees will continue to increase in coming years, costs must be controlled. Figure 1.2 illustrates the number of Medicare enrollees by year since 1989. Like the increased cost illustration, this graph clearly depicts the challenges and reasons for the impending changes.

FIGURE 1.2
NUMBER OF MEDICARE ENROLLEES BY YEAR

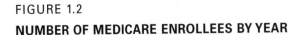

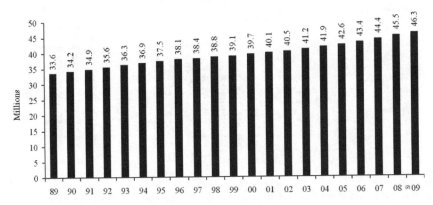

Source: Available at www.cms.hhs.gov/MedicareEnRpts/Downloads/HISMI05.pdf. Accessed January 13, 2011.

(1) *Hospital insurance (Part A) enrollees and/or Supplementary Medical Insurance (Part B) enrollees; includes all persons (aged and disabled).*
(2) *2008 figure reflects revised data obtained through e-mail correspondence.*

American Hospital Association, TrendWatch Chartbook 2010, Trends in the Overall Health Care Market, Chart 1.17. www.aha.org/aha/research-and-trends/chartbook/ch1.html. Accessed January 13, 2011.

Simply stated, our country is aging. The mass population of baby boomers now reaching retirement means a much greater number will be depending on government forms of reimbursement as opposed to private insurance. In addition, likely millions more are becoming subject to some form of healthcare through government or private insurance (previously the uninsured population within the United States), which will inevitably place unparalleled stress on the healthcare delivery system. This means costs must be controlled more than ever before. There are simply not enough dollars to go around in the next five to 10 years and beyond.

As the U.S. healthcare industry continues to grow in size and complexity, it is evident that there are significant variations in the quality of care (and to some extent how that care is delivered), and without question the cost of delivering it. All one has to do is compare the Medicare spending per enrollee across the nation to see huge variations, even though supposedly the same level of care is being rendered. These varied costs (and some outcomes) are not only true on a total absolute dollar basis within one locale; they flow to a per capita basis also. Further, this principle seems to apply across all levels of care and specialties. For example, the cost to deliver per capita for a cardiac patient is at varying levels, as is that for an orthopedic patient. Supposedly, Medicare has addressed this to some extent within its sustainable growth rate adjustment, which is regionalized and adjusted annually to consider these types of variations in care delivery and its cost. However, for the vast percentage of Medicare enrollees, provider reimbursement is based on a fee-for-service (FFS) payment structure that, while not indicting any particular provider for overuse, encourages the use of more services, more procedures, and overall higher charges.

Although a Medicare Advantage program covers roughly 30% of the Medicare enrollees and, as such, relies on private insurance companies representing this constituency, once again they are primarily based on a system that does not seem to align incentives, even though capitation payments to control use and costs largely exist within this program. In fact, in 2009, the Medicare Advantage program on a per-enrollee basis cost 114% more than FFS Medicare. Thus, even the Medicare Advantage program, under its capitation structure, has not held down costs or exhibited significant improvements in quality and outcomes.

Other possible solutions have been suggested that still would be largely FFS; they add on incentives for maintaining quality and controlling costs and, as such, focus on the specific areas where the need seems to be greatest. Although this is largely what the ACO reimbursement structure will entail, it has potential flaws.

Thus, as we consider the need for an ACO-type model, clearly we must get control of our costs while maintaining or improving the level of service and quality that results from such service. As we explore these payment mechanisms in detail, we consider the possibilities as well as how they would be administered and managed.

Basic ACO Tenets

Eligible providers

The final regulations have identified the types of providers who will be eligible to participate in an ACO entity. They include:

- Physicians

- Nurse practitioners

- Physician assistants

- Clinical nurse specialists

- Hospitals

- Other medical care providers/suppliers

Primary care providers (PCP) can participate with only one ACO during a contract period. The final CMS regulations added a provision that allows specialists who deliver the most number of primary care services to beneficiaries to be considered a PCP for assignment of Medicare beneficiaries to an ACO. In this type of situation, the specialist who was deemed to be a PCP due to the volume of primary care services rendered could only participate with one ACO during a contract period. Also, CMS liberalized the section on beneficiary assignment to include nurse practitioners (NP), physician assistants (PA), and clinical nurse specialists (CNS) as designated PCPs, thus limiting these providers to participation with only one CMS ACO during a given contract period. However, the other specialists have the ability to participate with multiple ACOs during a contract period.

ACOs most assuredly will include one or more hospitals; they also are likely to include nursing homes, ambulatory surgery centers, diagnostic centers, home healthcare, rehabilitation, and any or all entities enrolled in Medicare.

The primary characteristics of accountable care include the following:

- Clinical integration

- Coordination of care

- Costs and all other financial management

- Information technology (IT)

It is highly unlikely that any ACO will be successful—both initially and long-term—without these foundational characteristics. Moreover, they must have a solid infrastructure that is adequately represented by the various provider disciplines and specialties (e.g., hospitals, physicians, diagnostic centers, etc.). Sufficient access to capital is also a requirement in order to develop the infrastructure to support these four foundational characteristics. These key discussions will be the focus of following chapters in addition to exploring how an ACO would best establish these cornerstones.

ACO formation

ACOs will encompass provider groups that have established the functionality and infrastructure for making decisions relative to care and cost, but also are equipped to develop the capital, infrastructure, and reimbursement distributions, including bonus payments. These may include:

- Physician and other practitioners in private group practices

- Networks of practices, usually involving hospitals

- "Partnerships," "joint ventures," and/or other consortiums that qualify under antitrust and other regulations when involving hospitals and physicians. Foundations for these may include physician-hospital organizations (PHO), independent practice associations (IPA), and even management services organizations

- Fully integrated organizations, usually owned by hospitals where the provider physicians are employed or directly contracted through a professional services agreement

- Large consortiums of practitioners who are aligned in some manner that qualifies under antitrust restrictions; these could include physicians, nonphysician providers, nurses, therapists, and others

ACO qualifications

ACOs formed under the CMS program must meet at least the following criteria and have these features in place before they will be recognized by Medicare:

- Accountable for the overall care of their assigned Medicare beneficiaries

- Accept at least three years of participation (or a contract period, since those signing up in 2012 will have slightly more than three years in the first period)

- Be structured legally to allow shared savings to be distributed to providers based on certain performance criteria, not tied to volume (and also to handle loss allocation to provider participants under the Track 2 model)

- Entail sufficient numbers of primary care physicians to treat no less than 5,000 Medicare FFS beneficiaries

- Provide CMS with data and other information concerning PCPs and specialty care physicians participating in the ACO (as required by CMS)

- Develop and have in place working relationships for covering the patient population with a core group of specialty physicians

- Have an infrastructure of management and administration to oversee clinical and administrative systems

- Promote evidence-based medicine with specific processes in place

- Be equipped to report on quality and cost measures, plus be structured to coordinate care

- Be able to demonstrate "patient-centeredness," as defined by CMS

Financial ramifications

Following is a brief overview of bonuses and incentive payment opportunities:

- ACOs that demonstrate Medicare expenditures below established benchmarks are eligible for shared savings provided they meet the minimum savings rate and the quality requirements during the performance year

- CMS has finalized a sliding scale minimum savings rate (MSR) for Track 1 participants based on different sizes of ACOs (size is derived by number of beneficiaries assigned to an ACO)

- Those ACO entities who choose to participate under the Track 2 model will have a flat minimum savings rate of 2%

- Quality thresholds must be met by ACOs to earn incentive payments; these 33 measures have been outlined to be:

  - Care coordination/patient safety (six measures)

  - Patient/caregiver care experiences (seven measures)

  - Preventative health (eight measures)

  - At-risk population (12 measures)

Reporting requirements

CMS took into account many comments submitted in response to their proposed regulations regarding the hardship that some reporting requirements would cause. In response to these concerns, CMS attempted to reduce the amount of work required by participating providers in the submission of reporting information.

The 33 quality measures will be reported as outlined below in the final regulations:

- Seven measures will be collected via patient surveys

- Three measures will be calculated utilizing claim submission data

- One measure will be determined from the EHR Incentive Program data

- 22 measures will be collected via GPRO (Group Practice Reporting Option) Web interface

The Key Characteristics of Accountable Care

Earlier in this chapter, we briefly considered the foundational components of accountable care. Regardless of the ultimate regulations and overall requirements for establishing ACOs, it is apparent that these four cornerstones will be absolutely essential. Delving deeper, ACOs will have four foundational characteristics: clinical integration, coordination of care, engaging the patient, and a financial management system. A brief description of these aspects follows.

Clinical integration

Clinical integration, which is not new to provider organizations in concept, provides a conduit between various providers, with the capabilities to accumulate and exchange information to support and substantiate quality performance and outcomes. Clinically integrated provider organizations attempt to emphasize quality through their affiliation and therefore the ability to consolidate information and create improved standards of care. Ultimately, they use this data to measure their performance against such standards. With this knowledge, compliance is the norm. Further, education and overall improvements in operations result in better quality, which is the goal. Thus, the capacity for clinical integration supplants the ACO for functioning as the transforming entity within the healthcare delivery system.

Moreover, from a regulatory standpoint, clinical integration has been defined for some time by the U.S. government, and specifically the Federal Trade Commission. By definition, clinical integration requires provider organizations to improve efficiencies through monitoring and controlling quality service and costs. This is furthered through the selection of physician participant partners and employing evidence-based standards in the medical practice. Finally, to be successful in clinical integration, most believe a significant investment of both economic and human capital is essential, building the infrastructure largely through enhanced IT. For years, PHOs and IPAs that have not qualified to be more than messenger models to and from managed care payers are now capable of representing their constituent providers in joint contract negotiations with payers when they can demonstrate clinical integration. The anticipated plan for ACOs is to further the distinctiveness of PHOs/IPAs that are clinically integrated; thus, this clinically integrated entity will be used as a basis for the ACO—not only its existence, but its day-to-day functionality.

Coordination of care

A second consideration within the foundations of accountable care is the concept of care coordination. Our previous discussion on clinical integration is relevant to this in that the providers (through the ACO) must develop a system to coordinate care and thus exhibit a greater value in the care that is being provided. That is, providing the care at the right time, in the right place, at all times. Though a reasonable statement and common sense, this concept represents a significant change in today's healthcare delivery model. Care coordination in today's vernacular is more than just use management or simply aligning physicians into a common group or via contracting entities such as an IPA/PHO. It encompasses a patient-centric vision, and as such, changes will affect the way providers practice medicine. This will occur mostly in practice patterns for practicing medicine, plus new standards of information, management, and human resource skill sets.

Established physicians often find it difficult to change the way they practice. Although not inhibiting the formation of an ACO, organizations may face dramatic challenges wrought by required changes in the way the physicians think and practice. Helping physicians through education to understand evidence-based medicine principles and transcending these into day-to-day practice is a major challenge within this foundational characteristic and ultimately the success in forming and operating the ACO. Trying to work within a team to best understand the processes and other important characteristics of day-to-day care coordination is essential. Not surprisingly, this requires the organization (including the ACO) to carefully review and consider infrastructure, approach to care coordination programs, specific care coordination goals, and priorities in order to determine how best they can be effectively managed.

Engaging the patient

A critical component of care coordination going forward is empowering and engaging the patient. Educating patients and applying self-care concepts must be accomplished as a part of the overall care coordination plan. Patients who are engaged, well-informed, educated, and motivated to help treat their problem will result in a much stronger, more viable ACO. The proposed regulations further clarify this requirement by stating that communications must be easily understandable by patients, their family, and/or caregiver(s).

Another characteristic of ACO is a well-defined and managed operational infrastructure that will help ensure strong care coordination going forward. Finally, the organization that becomes a successful ACO and in turn provides good care coordination—the kind of care coordination that will be required—must have a well-defined and functional leadership and governance structure.

Regardless of how good the clinically-integrated and care-coordinated functions are, the ACO's success or failure will largely be based on its ability to collect, manage, share, and interpret information through technology processes. Health IT is nothing more than a support system for the members of the ACO to accumulate and disseminate the information and data. This quite simply cannot be done with any level of efficiency without automated healthcare technology. From historical performance, to future plans and budgets, to benchmarking against such standards—these are all a major part of the work toward an effective IT system within the ACO.

Financial management system

Finally, as with most or all entities of any size or makeup, a well-established and highly competent financial management system and staff will be necessary. Having the tools to support the financial modeling that will result is essential to establish ancillary or professional and/or hospital charges. The methodology of reimbursement will require very competent financial and managerial expertise. Likewise, a cost accounting and data collection system will be necessary to manage under the anticipated new payment models.

From a financial perspective, the ACO can move directly into working with the private/commercial payer community with this competency in place.

Thus, these foundations form the cornerstones of accountable care. Taking shortcuts in these areas would pose the risk of creating a less than functional entity.

Summary

The purpose of this overview is to outline the basic tenets of ACOs, to consider the overall characteristics and requirements, to explain how the reimbursement structure may work, and to explore proposed structure and infrastructure. In following chapters, the aspects presented in this overview are covered in detail. This should serve as a solid foundation for the reader—both in terms of considering the more detailed concepts in the remainder of the book and, most importantly, the ability to function in a healthcare environment that heavily includes ACOs.

How We Got Here

Like fashion cycles that seem to come and go every decade or so, healthcare seems to revolve by decade, moving from physician-hospital autonomy to physician-hospital alignment models, back and forth. Although each revolution is not an exact image of prior versions of collaboration, the cycle typically has some semblance of the old pattern but with new characteristics that address the current times and market (payer and patient) requirements. In healthcare, the changes that are now occurring are driven by and under the auspices of state and federal statutes via applicable regulatory bodies.

A Look Back at the 1980s and '90s

HMOs grew rapidly in the 1980s; by the mid-'90s, their market share was one-third of the large, commercially insured employer plans. This was partly due to the HMO act of 1973, which mandated employers with 25 or more employees to also offer a federally qualified HMO plan if they offered group health insurance to their staff. Furthermore, this law provided government subsidies to HMOs. The original concept of this type of managed care was to provide quality services to patients at a lower cost, with the emphasis on the primary care physician (PCP) to direct and manage the care of the patient. Typically, employers offered HMO coverage and the monthly premiums were the same for each member.

Employees were enticed by the HMO offerings of lower premiums, no deductibles, and coverage of routine/preventative care. During the '80s and for most of the '90s, preventative care (immunizations, physicals, checkups, etc.) was not usually covered by employers' standard group health insurance plans. Families with children typically enrolled in HMOs because it was financially beneficial for them—premiums were lower, immunizations and checkups were covered, and they ultimately had fewer out-of-pocket expenses. In return for the lower costs, members (the insured) were required to choose a PCP who was responsible for managing and directing the patient's care. The PCP was to focus on prevention of illnesses and management of chronic conditions to keep expenses at a minimum. The PCPs (family medicine, internal medicine, pediatricians, and, in some states, OB/GYNs), could only refer patients to specialists under the HMO's strict guidelines. Failure to follow the guidelines could result in a financial penalty to the PCP. The patients could not self-refer to a specialist, as they had to obtain a written referral from their PCP. Failure to obtain the referral could require the patient to pay for the specialists' services out of his or her own pocket.

Specialists also contracted with HMOs and were reimbursed under a reduced fee-for-service schedule. Many HMOs withheld a percentage of scheduled payments from participating providers as part of a "quality" pool. If the plan was profitable and delivered quality care to the patients, the HMO would share the pool with the physicians and reimburse them the amounts fully or partially due under their schedules. One measure of quality of care (and profitability) was managing the number of inpatient hospital days. HMOs around the country had staff devoted to hospital discharge planning and the reduction in the number of "bed-days" (a day in which a patient is hospitalized overnight) per month. Physicians and hospitals participated in the HMO networks—not due to the possibility of receiving better reimbursements, but because large employers controlled the healthcare markets and the providers could not afford to lose their patient base (employees of these medium to large corporations).

There were two predominant models of HMOs: the staff model and the independent practice association (IPA). The IPA was the most common model across the country, but it did vary by geographical location. For example, in California (home of the oldest HMO in the country, Kaiser Permanente, circa 1945), staff models were more predominant. An IPA HMO contracts with private physicians (and hospitals) to provide services to the HMO members. The providers can treat HMO and non-HMO members in their clinics and facilities. PCPs typically received a flat monthly fee called *capitation* from the HMO for each member (i.e., per member per month). That fee was paid to the PCP regardless of whether the patient visited the physician and without respect to the number of visits the patient made to the PCP. Some physicians received monthly payments for patients who never required treatment and greatly profited from these healthy patients. Other providers had to manage the care of chronic or frequent-visiting patients, which cost more money than they received under their monthly capitation fees. In the capitation environment, physicians have greater profitability with fewer patient visits. In a fee-for-service environment, a physician's revenue increases with greater numbers of visits.

A staff model HMO (also known as a closed panel) has employed physicians, and those physicians can only treat members of the HMO. The HMO owns practices that serve their members for both primary and specialty care. Depending on the HMO, the patient may not always be able to see the same PCP for each visit. This has caused dissatisfaction with patients as they want the consistency of seeing the same physician, and they desire the ability to choose which doctor provides care to them. Kaiser, the largest managed care system in the country, is a staff model HMO. As of December 2009, Kaiser had nearly 8 million members and employed over 15,000 physicians. With its foundation in the '40s, Kaiser has proven to be a successful HMO-managed system.

The Alternatives to HMOs

Even though HMOs were growing during the '80s, some parts of the country did not embrace this type of managed care; even where HMOs were common, large employers were looking for alternative medical plans to reduce their costs while keeping their employees happy. Most large employers are self-insured for group insurance, which saves them large premiums. They pay premiums for reinsurance to cover high-dollar claims and catastrophic amounts over a certain limit outlined in their agreement with the third-party insurance administrator. Insurance companies were also looking for ways to reduce payments as the cost of medical claims continued to grow at high rates during the period. As discussed, HMOs require members to receive treatment only from approved HMO physicians, and all members must follow strict rules. If the insured member fails to obtain a referral from his or her PCP to a specialist, or if the member obtains primary care treatment outside of his or her HMO network, no benefits are available and the patient must pay for this care. Some people found these HMO rules too restrictive and did not enroll or re-enroll in HMOs. By staying in or moving to a traditional indemnity health plan, they paid higher premiums. It also cost their employer more for this coverage and it was more costly for the insurance carriers to administer.

Preferred provider organization model

The preferred provider organization (PPO) emerged in the early '80s. A PPO is an organization that has an agreement between a group or network of providers and a third-party payer. The legal entity of a PPO can be provider sponsored, employer organized, or managed by a third-party payer (insurance company). Most PPOs were created by insurance companies and/or large employers as a means to reduce healthcare costs and expenses.

Participants in PPOs are typically employees covered by their employers' group insurance plans. The PPO plans offer premiums higher than an HMO but less expensive than a traditional insurance plan. Most PPOs also provide limited preventative care coverage and require small copayments for physician visits. Unlike HMOs, certain types of services under a PPO are subject to an annual deductible and coinsurance payment by the patient. However, the attracting PPO feature over an HMO is that the patient can see any doctor he or she chooses. If the physician is part of the PPO network, benefits are paid under the higher PPO benefit levels. If the patient visits a non-PPO physician or hospital, they receive benefits at a reduced level, thus incurring greater out-of-pocket expenses, but expenses that are less than if they were in an HMO and chose to go outside of the network physicians and rules. Preferred provider networks grew substantially in the '90s and currently are one of the most common types of plans offered in the 2000s.

Point of service model

Point of service (POS) models followed in the footsteps of PPOs in the early '90s. POS is a hybrid of HMO and PPO provisions. Some people call a POS an "HMO without walls." The concept of POS health plans is to offer managed care at a reasonable price, with limited network benefits, while providing some choices to patients. Under a POS plan, the patient must choose a PCP who is responsible for managing the patient's care. The PCP, when necessary, should direct patients to specialists within the POS network to help ensure continuity of care and cost containment. However, a patient may choose to go outside of the POS physician or hospital network. Doing so will result in greatly reduced benefits for the charges incurred by nonparticipating providers. A POS gives a patient the benefits of lower costs and greater services similar to an HMO, but the flexibility to go outside of the network with some reimbursement options.

Medicare Prospective Payment System

In 1983, the federal government introduced the prospective payment system (PPS) for Medicare hospitalizations. The goal of the new payment methodology was to change hospital behavior through financial incentives that encourage more cost-efficient management of medical care. Under PPS, hospitals are paid a predetermined rate for each Medicare admission. Each patient admission is classified into a diagnosis-related group (DRG) on the basis of clinical information at the time of admission. The final DRG classification may be amended at the time of discharge depending on outliers or other extenuating factors. However, typically, the original DRG is retained. Under the DRG payment model, the hospital is paid a flat rate for the DRG, regardless of the actual services provided. If the hospital treats a high percentage of low-income patients, it receives a percentage add-on payment applied to the DRG-adjusted base payment rate. This add-on, known as the disproportionate share hospital adjustment, provides for a percentage increase in Medicare payment for hospitals that qualify under either of two statutory formulas designed to identify hospitals that serve a disproportionate share of low-income patients. For qualifying hospitals, the amount of this adjustment may vary based on the outcome of the statutory calculation. Also, if the hospital is an approved teaching hospital, it receives a percentage add-on payment for each case paid through inpatient PPS. This add-on, known as the indirect medical education adjustment, varies depending on the ratio of residents-to-beds under the PPS for operating costs and according to the ratio of residents-to-average daily census under the PPS for capital costs.

For particular cases that are unusually costly, known as outlier cases, the inpatient PPS payment is increased.

The Centers for Medicare & Medicaid Services (CMS) uses separate PPSs for reimbursement to acute inpatient hospitals, home health agencies, hospice, hospital outpatient, inpatient psychiatric facilities, inpatient rehabilitation facilities, long-term care hospitals, and skilled nursing facilities. Some PPS reimbursements are based upon a flat DRG and some are a per diem. Over time, 21 states adopted similar PPS models for Medicaid, and some third-party payers adopted DRGs for some of their HMOs and PPOs, including outpatient or same-day surgeries.

The implementation of a flat payment (DRG) to the hospital changed the relationship between physicians and hospitals in the '80s. Hospitals found themselves reaching out to physicians in an attempt to get them to help reduce the length of stay. Yet the attending physician was acting on behalf of the patient and the perceived belief that a longer confinement would improve the patient's recovery. And, in direct conflict with the hospital's DRG reimbursement, the physicians were reimbursed in a manner that incentivized more care (more inpatient visits) resulting in greater reimbursement to the attending physicians. This caused some friction and challenges between to the two diverse caregivers. In hopes of staying financially viable, hospitals attempted to balance the new payment model with early patient discharges and that created additional challenges between hospitals and physicians.

Although not part of the Medicare PPS, the federal government did recognize the need to curtail reimbursements to physicians. In 1992, Medicare introduced the resource-based relative value scale (RBRVS) as a basis for physician payments. This methodology changed payments based on physician charges to a fee schedule to reduce Medicare expenditures due to budget concerns. The RBRVS fee schedule was part of the Omnibus Budget Reconciliation Act of 1989.

Physician-Hospital Organizations

Physician-hospital organizations (PHO) initially emerged in the '80s in response to the DRG payments under Medicare's PPS. They served as a means to provide incentives to physicians to help reduce inpatient costs. As managed care grew in the '80s and '90s, PHOs expanded. Hospital PHO members wanted to improve their contracting positions with managed care organizations, as well as facilitate collaborative efforts with physicians. This type of alliance put hospitals in partnership with physicians to negotiate packaged rates with purchasers. The PHO became one of the first forms of cooperative alignment without employment contracts between physicians in private practices and hospitals.

Across the country, the success of PHOs varied by organization. Some appeared to be highly successful, while others faltered with poor management and lack of execution of plans. As capitation payments to physicians declined, PHOs dissolved. However, several hundred still exist. In Atlanta, the DeKalb PHO comprises of DeKalb Medical Center (a 525-bed facility) and more than 500 private practice physicians. This PHO, which has been in existence since 2003, claims that it has improved quality of care by delivering better outcomes, reduced costs, and fewer unnecessary tests through the use of evidence-based medicine that member physicians agree on. It is perceived by some that they have established the basis for an ACO with the success of their PHO.

Summary

Those who have been in the healthcare industry for more than 25 years saw monumental changes in the 1980s that included increased strength by managed care organizations, the introduction of Medicare's PPS and DRGs, development of PPO and POS plans, and several other changes that affected provider reimbursement and the care given to patients. Many of the changes also affected the patient's financial responsibility by requiring greater out-of-pocket payments.

When physicians and hospitals were forced to "play in the sandbox" together due to the emergence of DRGs and PHOs, those situations did not always work well. Theoretically, they cooperated because it was in both of their best interests from an economic perspective. However, physicians withdrew as quickly as they could when it was financially feasible. Most physicians in the '90s preferred the autonomy of their private practice without alignment with a hospital. Now, with cuts in physician reimbursements, physicians are gravitating back to the hospital alignment models, some "at arm's length" through directorships or co-management arrangements. Others are moving into full alignments and becoming hospital employees in order to survive financially.

Under the 2010 Patient Protection and Affordable Care Act, Congress created provisions for voluntary ACOs, as described in Chapter 1. Physicians and hospitals will have the option to participate in these organizational models based on certain criteria. The final CMS ACO regulations indicate that physicians and hospitals will need to be aligned closely in order to reduce costs, improve patient care, and produce evidence-based results. In addition, the financial savings will be paid to the ACO entity if quality guidelines are met while bringing total costs below a certain threshold. The ACO will then "share" (distribute) the savings to the participating providers. The shared savings and quality programs are explained in Chapters 8 and 10, respectively, of this book. The future alignment of physicians and hospitals will require extensive information technology integration and all-embracing collaboration in order to render success in patient-centered ACOs. This collaboration appears that it will far exceed the demands of any previous partnership under HMOs, PHOs, or other earlier models.

What We Anticipate About the Accountable Care Concept

As history has shown, payers have few tools to impact the cost of care. Discounting, their most frequently used approach, has little impact on use—it may actually encourage more—and at some point will meet provider resistance. Diagnosis-related groups (DRG), capitation, case rates, per diems, and similar strategies were an attempt to shift the cost containment responsibility to providers. Although the concept was a good one, the models were flawed and ineffective. None of the strategies addressed the total care cost, and certainly none addressed the quality of the care delivered. The emphasis now is on accountable care as a total concept. This chapter focuses on the general characteristics of accountable care, specifically as it relates to accountable care organizations (ACO).

Accountable Care Organizations

The most recent attempt to hold the line on healthcare costs is the ACO. The theory is to provide financial incentives to broadly integrated care networks to reduce the total cost of care for a defined population while improving the quality and efficiency of the care delivered. The payer will share the savings from the lower costs with the provider network. This is nothing new. The concept is based on capitation models that have been around for decades. The health reform plan proposed by President Clinton in the early 1990s has provider networks that are very similar to those in the new reform law. The renewed interest is driven by Medicare's current unsustainability and the government's inability to make benefit reductions that are both politically acceptable and financially significant. The result is to shift that problem to the provider. States that face critical financial issues will find the approach appealing for their Medicaid populations, and it is certain that commercial payers will want to lower their costs so they are more attractive to their employer customers.

Although it is definite that an ACO, to be successful, will need sophisticated clinical and financial data systems and the financial strength to create the care environment necessary to provide services to its defined population, it is also sure that there will need to be a culture in which the ACO can thrive. This culture will require that hospitals share control with physicians, that physicians agree to adopt standards of care that may be different from what they have traditionally provided, and that all components of the ACO work collaboratively to provide quality care in an efficient manner.

Why ACOs?

The 2010 Medicare Trustee Report to Congress states that the Health Insurance Trust Fund, the money used to support Part A of Medicare, began to spend more than it took in during 2008, and projects that the Health Insurance Trust Fund is scheduled for depletion in 2017 if nothing changes. The impact of the reform law was not factored. Parts B and D, in theory, are supported by premiums paid by participants; however, the annual changes to the physician fee schedule create an unsustainable financial picture because the premiums assume that the 30% reduction in physician fees took place as required by existing law.

Some questions exist about whether the fee-for-service (FFS) environment creates inefficiencies in the delivery of care. Data repeatedly reflect wide differences in the total cost for similar procedures in different geographic markets without significant differences in outcomes. The January 2011 Medicare Payment Advisory Commission (MedPAC) report to the congress titled "Regional Variation in Medicare Service Use" documented that procedures such as imaging vary by 30% for similar patient populations between geographic regions after correcting for differences in patient demographics and regional costs service; use by beneficiaries can vary by 30%, depending on where they live; and the average monthly cost can vary by more than 50%. Service use by patients who died during the year of study was nine times higher than those that did not, and the use by the decedents followed the same use patterns as non-decedents in the same market; higher-use markets provided more care per person in both cases. Similar but larger differences were seen in other care sectors, such as post-acute care. These data did not correlate with high indices of health. Cost does not drive quality.[1]

Large integrated systems, such as the Mayo Clinic, are able to "package price" procedures based on their efforts to standardize care and track costs. Once cost and outcomes become more predictable, the ACO can better estimate the total cost of caring for a defined population and establish appropriate incentives.

"Health, United States, 2010," a publication of the Centers for Disease Control and Prevention, reported that treatment related to chronic conditions accounts for approximately 75% of total healthcare expenditures and that expenditures by Medicare and Medicaid have increased nearly 10% annually since 1990. Nationally, we spend more than $8,000 annually per person on healthcare services.[2]

Given these facts, it is clear that the current approach to financing care does not have a positive impact on either cost or quality. As long as the total cost of providing care is less than the amount of revenue produced by the care, there is no mandate for anyone to look further at cost containment, other than improvement of profit. If physicians and others avoid being sued for malpractice, quality is adequate. Regional cost differences are addressed by regional payment differences, often unrelated to the actual cost profile of that region.

The basic theory behind the potential benefit of the ACO model is that those individuals with the most knowledge of what is needed to maintain health, physicians, will take a leadership role on managing the total care process and will be proactive in improving patient compliance with those steps that have proven to avoid or lessen the impacts from diseases and chronic conditions. Many studies have shown the financial result of obesity, smoking, uncontrolled hypertension and diabetes, routine screening, cardiovascular exercise, and others. The ACO, through its physician members, would track patient behaviors and identify potential risks so that additional resources can be employed before more expensive interventions are needed.

At the same time, other procedures, such as expensive surgeries, might be made less costly if supplies, medications, in-hospital care, rehabilitation, and similar components could be standardized. If these items were common among all of the physicians, performing the procedure differences in outcomes would be much easier to study and "quality" would be easier to measure.

The ACO, if it is to deliver on its promise, will need to focus attention on how to maintain the health of its members' patients with chronic conditions, educate patients and perhaps provide incentives related to need for preventive care and personal care, and find ways to reduce the cost of the most expensive procedures in its market. At the same time, the ACO will need to create the ability to compare outcomes with the provider network and between the ACO and other markets. It is highly unlikely that acute primary care will change dramatically; however, it will be important for the ACO to find ways to deliver care in non-emergency department settings and perhaps have appropriate care delivered by nonphysician providers, such as nurse practitioners and physician assistants.

What Will an ACO Look Like?

It is unlikely that one ACO model will work in all settings. With the release of the final rule, we know what the Centers for Medicare & Medicaid Services (CMS) ACOs should look like; however, we anticipate that they may change during 2013 based upon the first year's results. Also, private ACOs have taken many shapes in 2010 and 2011. The ultimate design will be influenced by the ACO sponsor, the provider capabilities in the specific market, the patient population that joins the ACO, and the type of cost-reduction incentives that are provided. Common model characteristics include being patient-centered, focusing on quality, having a new focal point of care, being innovative, maintaining technological savvy, and staying value driven. Brief descriptions follow.

Patient-centered

The ACO will need to make the patient a partner in his or her care. It is critical for the "accountability" in the ACO to be tied to the needs of the patient and not to the payer or the provider. Although the ACO will need to provide a win-win environment for all of the components, it will succeed only if the patient perceives that the ACO provides a benefit that was not true of his or her former FFS care environment. The medical home model is a good example of how changes in the way care is delivered can change these perceptions. It is likely that patients will have expanded access to provider contacts through phone consultations and perhaps e-mail. Primary care practices will assume an active role in helping patients maneuver the care system and will collect and study the results of specialty and hospital encounters. This is really the gatekeeper HMO concept, but rather than an obstacle to getting care desired, the ACO will need to help the patient understand the value of the physician partner. It is anticipated that primary care practices and/or ACO entities will further expand the roles of physician extenders (nurse practitioners and physician assistants) to act as liaisons and care coordinators to provide better accessibility for the patient.

Some ACOs may opt to include patient representatives in their governance structure in either an advisory or policy role. The federally supported community health center program requires that grantees include "users" (actual patients of the center) on the governing body. The CMS ACO regulations require that a beneficiary participate as a member of the governing body (see Chapter 7 for specific details regarding this provision).

At present, Medicare ACOs will allow patients to opt out if they wish and rejoin the traditional Medicare model, so patient satisfaction will be a key component.

The demise of the gatekeeper HMO was due, in part, to the pushback from patients; so, again, the ACO will have clear incentives to maintain a patient-centric environment if they wish to succeed.

Quality-focused

Restricting care is always a risky strategy. "Death panel" rumors during the debate about the health reform legislation underscore the public perception that less care is always bad. ACOs will be challenged to better manage the care of member-patients while assuring that care is both appropriate and of high quality, even when the definition of quality may be under debate. Evidence-based care will be the cornerstone of the ACO. What has worked well in other settings will be the gold standard for care. Quality, however, will need to be matched with efficiency. Access to care will be critical, and movement through the care continuum will require the cooperation of all components. A patient's perception of quality is far different from that of a provider. A patient who has had an unpleasant encounter with a front desk receptionist, a long wait time, a gruff technician, or a disinterested physician will be hard to convince that the care received really is of high quality. Providers will need to balance the patient perception with the clinical care.

Quality will need to be tracked, with incentives and disincentives tied to the results. Providers that cannot meet the quality standards will need to be removed from the care network. This is critical, both from a promise that will need to be made to patients, as well as the cost of poor quality. This will be especially difficult in physician networks. Historically, there has been significant latitude in how physicians and patients interact and what care is deemed appropriate. Physician leadership will need to be willing to engage their peers in frank discussions of quality and quality shortcomings. Finally, quality findings will need to be shared with member-patients so that they understand that, although their care environment is different from what they have traditionally experienced, it is likely providing care at a high or higher level.

Many organizations currently collect and report data related to quality indicators, but reporting is far different from using those data to make functional changes in how care is delivered and who delivers it. This element may have a steep learning curve for many providers.

New focal point of care

ACOs will need to move away from the episodic acute care that has become the norm in an FFS environment and create proactive systems that remind patients of the need for preventive services, actively manage their diseases, and educate them about how they can play an active role in their health. Our historic system has not rewarded this new approach because payments were tied only to illness episodes or perhaps annual preventive visits. The ACO will need to find ways to compensate providers for the following:

- Time and effort involved in responding to telephone questions that may avoid an office encounter

- Actively monitoring chronic patients to assure that they receive the supportive care they need in the time period they need it

- Collecting data on care across many settings to assure that none of the interventions has a negative impact on another (such as drug interactions)

- Ensuring that providers or staff are available to educate the patient about his or her problem, treatment, and any behavioral changes that may lessen or avoid problems in the future

Collecting and sharing clinical data across many settings is another new experience for many providers. Access to hospital data often means that physicians receive paper reports or need to access a data system different from the one used in their office. Many times, not all the data makes its way into the patient record because that is a time-consuming and costly process. Data sharing across the care continuum will be required.

Preventing illness will be preferred over treating illness. If a specialist never sees a patient, the cost of care will benefit. If a hospitalization is avoided, the ACO may well share in the savings. It will be critical to differentiate between withholding care and providing care in the most appropriate manner. The former cannot be allowed, and the latter must be encouraged. The successful ACO will encourage the orthopedist to teach the family physician how to manage nonsurgical musculoskeletal issues and be rewarded for reducing the number of referrals. Physicians will take a closer look at clinical indicators before they resort to expensive and perhaps unnecessary diagnostic procedures. Aggressive care in the office or home may replace the need to admit the patient to the hospital.

Innovative

The ACO model requires that care providers do something that really has not been done before, certainly not on a large scale. Although some point to the integrated models of the Mayo Clinic, Cleveland Clinic, Geisinger Health System, and others, the ACO initiative requires that organizations that have not had the decades of culture and system building acquired by these providers attempt to replicate their success. Innovation will be required in the integration of different provider cultures and the egos that accompany those cultures; it will be necessary in the development and use of clinical data systems, and it will be required in the financial arena, as well. Details as finite as who will get paid and what savings are to be shared and as broad as what providers are selected to become a part of the ACO itself will require innovative thinking and action.

Is it likely that a group of open-minded individuals sitting around a planning table will create a viable ACO without problems? This is doubtful. This means that the process itself must be both deliberate and careful and all players must be committed to the eventual model. Unless the group is open to dramatic change, many obstacles will arise that can derail the process. It may be far easier to create the technical environment than the cultural one. Data systems can be made to communicate, compensation models and cost-capture programs can do what is needed, but it will take time and effort for physicians, hospital leadership, and ancillary care providers to move away from their protective turf issues and agree that care will be delivered where and how it makes the most sense, regardless of who "wins."

Technologically savvy

No ACO will succeed unless it is supported by a robust data environment that collects both clinical and cost data and then makes it available for use by others within the ACO. In some cases, the ACO will decide that it also wants to process and pay the claims submitted for the care provided, which will require additional technology. How these systems will need to work is addressed later in the chapter, but what is key is that the technology must be used, and it must be used in a similar manner by all. ACOs cannot tolerate physicians that choose to dictate notes rather than use the electronic health record (EHR); they cannot allow hospitals to have data systems that do not move information to the system in physician offices; they cannot require that entries be made separately into multiple data systems or that data need to be retrieved from multiple systems.

The private ACO will need to collect revenue and make payments to providers, so it will function much like the insurance plan with which it partners. Few providers already have this capability. The cost of technology should not be underestimated. In many instances, current systems will simply be unable to provide the support needed by the ACO. The choice will be to not become an ACO, borrow a data system from an ACO and simply be a network member, or invest in new systems.

Value-driven

The concept behind the creation of an ACO is the premise that it can deliver high-quality care at a cost that is less than the current expense. This proposition requires that providers examine the current care process and identify those services that do not beneficially contribute to the ultimate outcome. This might include tests that, in some or all cases, could be avoided, care settings that might be appropriate and less costly, approaches to treatment that differ from those in the local market but have proven effective in other regions, and inclusion of providers that have proven their efficiency and cost-effectiveness.

This value foundation will require that an ACO have the ability to capture the cost of care (not charges) so that these data can be compared to outcomes. The public will want to know that, in return for accepting more stringent rules about how they consume care, the overall care process is being monitored to assure that it remains appropriate. The providers within an ACO will want to be able to identify areas that require further cost controls so that they can share in larger pools of savings.

Structural Change

A private ACO will likely be a new entity that exists only to provide the support services needed by the ACO. These services will include the collection and dissemination of revenue from payers, the collection and analysis of use and cost data from the network providers, the development and maintenance of the contracting relationships among the various ACO provider participants, and the monitoring of quality indicators and the enforcement of quality standards. The ACO entity will likely not own or manage the data systems that support the ACO, except for financial systems, but will use data that it obtains from those systems to make operational decisions.

What will change is how the various components of an ACO interact. Physicians will be tasked with making decisions and setting standards about how care will be delivered and what treatments are most appropriate and efficient. These decisions will be based on the experience of the ACO physicians and data obtained from more mature managed care environments. What is decided will then be implemented, not only by the physicians but also the departments within the hospital, and by the ancillary care providers within the ACO. The physicians will not manage the hospital or ancillary facility, yet their decisions will have an impact on how those resources function.

Physicians that have made demands about what products are stocked by hospitals or how units are staffed will need to gain approval from the ACO if their desires differ from the standards that are developed. Hospital leaders will be able to shrug their shoulders, point to the ACO, and tell the physician how they would like to honor that request, but that may not be the best solution.

Hospitals will likely contribute technical expertise in information technology (IT), finance, materials management, perhaps payer contracting, and capital. How each of those components functions, however, will be the decision of the ACO.

Complicating this entire process will be the reality that many patients seen by the ACO providers will not be covered by the ACO. They will be traditional FFS patients that will carry with them the same behavioral inducements that have brought the healthcare system to this point. Care decisions may well be made based on the health plan rather than the clinical picture. Whereas it is unlikely that patients will be tattooed with "ACO" to assure cost-effective treatment, the success or failure of the ACO may be tied to the percentage of patients that it represents. Will provider behavior truly change if only some of the patients are from the ACO model? Large independent physician association (IPA) networks in California have seen economic success because the vast majority of patients seen by the providers have the same financial incentives and disincentives.

What all this means is that the greatest change may well need to be psychological rather than functional. If a substantial percentage of the patient base is represented by ACO members, the providers will become accustomed to the sharing of information, the coordination of care, and the collaborative sharing of financial resources. This will strengthen over time. If the ACO model fails to gain wide acceptance in the market, it is likely that the ACO will not produce meaningful savings to make the model attractive to providers, and the project may fail.

Also changing will be how funds flow through the care system. It is unlikely that there will be one approach that will work in all ACOs. What will be common is the fact that the ACO will be the contracting agency with the payer, public or private, and all funds will be received by the ACO and then distributed to the component providers. Depending on the size of the private ACO, this may require a sophisticated claims processing capability. Smaller organizations may contract this service to either the payer or some administrative services organization similar to those used by self-insured employers.

If you think about structure as you would an organizational chart, the ACO will be at the top and the hospital, physicians, and ancillary services will "work" for the ACO (see Figure 3.1). Payment and care policies will be developed at the ACO level, and payment models will be determined by the ACO. This makes it critical that all components of the ACO be a part of the policy-setting process so that none of the critical participants feels that they are at a disadvantage. This would cripple collaboration.

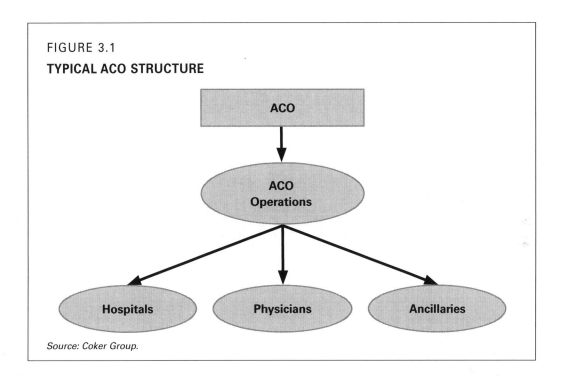

FIGURE 3.1
TYPICAL ACO STRUCTURE

Source: Coker Group.

In some markets, a dominant medical group or network of medical groups may be the formative agent and simply contract with hospitals for their services. This is common in the markets served by the large California IPAs. Although we can anticipate that hospitals will play a leading role in ACO formation and operation, these alternative structures may appear as diagramed in Figure 3.2.

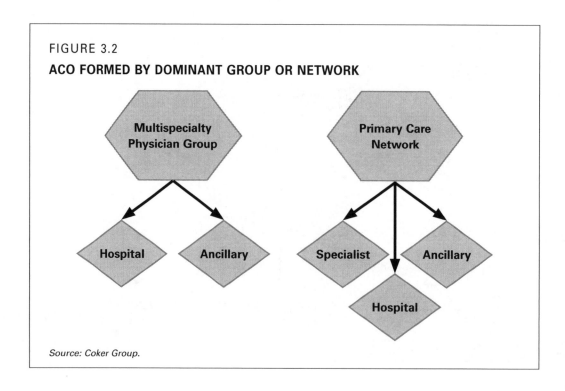

FIGURE 3.2

ACO FORMED BY DOMINANT GROUP OR NETWORK

Source: Coker Group.

Challenges of Collaboration

Many participants in an ACO are currently competitors and operate in a win-lose environment. How then, do you undo years of experience and create an environment of collaboration? Not easily. Specialists depend on referrals from primary care physicians (PCP) and direct access from more sophisticated patients. Gatekeeper model HMOs were never a favorite of the specialist. Hospitals depend on admissions from physicians, typically the specialists. Once the patient is admitted, the hospital either hopes the physician is efficient (Medicare DRG) or less so (per diem payments). Ancillary providers, such as freestanding imaging centers, often compete directly with hospitals and often at a lower cost, which referring physicians really do not care about. Patients may care, but that depends on their insurance plan.

Hospitals are happy to get the admissions from the physicians, but they do not appreciate interference in how their units are run, how their staffing is managed, and what they purchase. Physicians and hospitals know little about how the other is paid; however, physicians know that they send business to hospitals and ancillary providers with nothing in return.

Unless the rules change, these players have little incentive to cooperate, let alone collaborate. The ACO concept promises to change the rules. Physicians, as a group, need to standardize care and determine the resources needed to deliver that care. They can do this on their own, or they can adopt evidence-based best practices from others. Once adopted, these standards need to be communicated to downstream providers so that they know what services will be demanded and what supplies and staff will be required. Physicians may need to participate in the training of clinical support staff to ensure that care standards are met, regardless of the setting.

Hospitals and ancillary providers will need to cede control to the physicians as they decide on care models, resources, and staff requirements. It is almost certain that, if an ACO functions as intended, use of hospital resources (and ancillary services) will decline. What, then, is the motivation for these providers to participate? Using care standards will make the care requirements more predictable and, as a result, the resources more predictable. This will allow better management of capacity and costs. Additionally, if an admission or an image is avoided, the savings will be divided by the ACO providers as a group. Hospitals will be rewarded for not providing a service. Specialists will be rewarded for not getting a referral, and they avoid the costs associated with that visit.

In theory, all providers will benefit from a successful ACO, and, as a result, there are reasons that they should work with their colleagues in the development of the most efficient system possible. The need for each component may diminish, which may reduce the total number of specialists, imaging centers, or beds that are needed. However, those providers that remain will likely be more fully used and that use will be more predictable. Management should be able to improve operating margins as a result. This will reduce the cost of each service even more.

Although this sounds like a compelling argument for collaboration, it will require overcoming years of distrust, competition, and isolation. Previously, we mentioned that the psychological barriers may be more difficult to overcome than the technical. Collaboration will be the battleground.

Clinical integration

What does the term "clinical integration" mean? Physicians will work for hospitals? One entity provides the total spectrum of care? The answer can vary from all of these to none of them. Likely, the ACO model will differ from market to market. Clinical integration will refer to the ability of the various ACO components (hospitals, physicians, others) to jointly plan how care can best be provided and develop methods for tracking and measuring quality and cost.

Integration will include seamless sharing of clinical data, a common health record for each patient so care decisions can be based on a full knowledge of the total clinical picture. It will also include open discussion between providers so that the needs of the patient can be managed at the least expensive and most appropriate site of care. If physicians and home care providers can devise a care program that avoids hospitalization, everyone wins, including the patient.

Clinical integration does not mean that all of the various physician specialties need to be part of the same group or that the physicians must be part of a practice network owned by the hospital. Integration is not structural; it is conceptual and operational.

A good example of integration might be a recent experience by a patient with back pain. Unsure about what was wrong, the patient tried a program of exercise without benefit. In fact, the pain got worse. The patient then saw a PCP who offered a number of medications but indicated that the patient would need to be seen by the orthopedist. No diagnostic studies were ordered because the specialist would want to make his or her own decisions about that. When the patient finally got to see the specialist, weeks later, a simple x-ray revealed a disc problem that was aggravated by the exercise. Integration would have provided a means for the patient to initially contact a physician to ask if exercise was appropriate, may have been told to get the x-ray, and the problem would have been discovered before any more damage was done. Inappropriate medications could have been avoided, visits to physicians could have been reduced (or eliminated), and the time spent by the physicians could have been directed at those that needed their care more appropriately.

If this model is expanded to the care of a large population, the potential cost savings could be significant. In our example, what if a MRI had been ordered, or physical therapy, or the patient tried other specialists? The costs would have been substantially higher with the same outcome.

In our clinical example in the ACO environment, the patient would feel comfortable in an early physician contact, because there would be no financial barrier. Further, the physicians would welcome the contact, because they could better manage the needs of the patient.

Ultimately, clinical integration will accomplish the following:

- Provide a vehicle, and a reward, for physicians to help hospitals improve operational efficiency at the unit level through staff training and standardization

- Provide incentives to quickly move patients to the most appropriate site of care without concerns for lost revenue

- Align the incentives of:

    - The patient (get better)

    - The hospital (predict resource needs)

    - The physician (benefit from active patient management)

    - Others (access to patient population)

Healthcare information technology

Whereas the topic of health IT (HIT) will receive a more thorough focus in Chapter 11, our focus here is what changes will be needed in preparation for ACOs and not how technology functions.

Just as meaningful use raised awareness of the role of EHRs and the sales of software, the ACO will make robust data systems a requirement for success. It will be critical that ACOs not only have fully functional clinical and financial data systems but that all users understand how they must use them and comply with those use requirements.

Although a growing number of medical practices have adopted an EHR, few routinely share electronic data with the hospital or other agencies. That data sharing is usually through access to another software system or receipt of an electronic fax document into the EHR. (The electronic fax is non-discrete data and thus cannot be integrated into the patient's record for reporting and searching—it can only be read as a document image.) The ACO concept is based on a universal health record that collects and stores all of the information on a patient, regardless of the site of care, and makes those data available as needed to guide the future care of the patient. What the cardiologist prescribed during a recent hospitalization will be available to the family physician during the annual preventive visit. The emergency department physician will have the full picture of the patient as they assess the problem that brought them to the emergency room and will be guided by the care that others provided.

Because data systems must be used to be effective, a focus will be on the ease of use and degree of appropriateness in multiple settings. The system that was developed by a physician-specialist and his or her programmer friend that is sold to other similar specialists may not have a bright future unless it can seamlessly move data to the umbrella repository and retrieve the data needed by the specialist user. Hospitals that use multiple specialized clinical programs will need to ensure that they can all communicate with each other as well as with those systems outside the hospital. Other than getting physicians, hospitals, and others to work collaboratively, HIT integration may be the most challenging aspect of ACO development. It will certainly be the most expensive.

Health systems that have begun to move down the integration pathway are reporting IT expenses of tens of millions, if not hundreds of millions of dollars over the course of their journey. Many hospitals and health systems function as silos when it comes to their clinical systems. Laboratory systems may or may not interface with the physician EMR, and cardiac diagnostic systems my not electronically forward results to the specialist. The oncology research software may not link to anything. All this will need to change.

Organizations will need to make a hard decision related to the cost of creating multiple data interfaces and the likelihood of a workable outcome versus the adoption of a new system with proven interoperability. Significant historic investments may no longer have value. If new systems are the choice, then training and learning curve issues become important.

It is also likely that vendors will suggest that their system is the absolute answer to every situation. Senior leadership will need to depend on clinical and IT professionals (and perhaps independent, highly qualified HIT consultants) to evaluate those claims and provide the best recommendations about what needs to be adopted and what is unlikely to be of benefit. This will stretch existing resources, as everyone still needs to support the current HIT environment and care for the patients who are now seeking care. Workgroups will need to be formed, time and resources allocated, and clear outcomes defined.

In some cases, organizations will be moving toward compliance with meaningful use requirements only to learn that, as the ACO develops, their data system no longer fits into the overall data environment. This will certainly result in lost time and effort and may well end up in lost revenue. Even if organizations ultimately decide that an ACO does not fit into their strategic vision, the time and effort spent in a reexamination of the current data systems will be well spent. The cost of either not having access to data or moving data manually through the system will become more of a burden as reimbursement in the non-ACO world results in ever-thinning margins.

The final challenge that we will face is the need for our financial systems to extract data from our clinical systems. The successful ACO will have the ability to aggregate costs into care episodes and then compare those episodes across providers and settings, as well as against normative data obtained elsewhere. This is vastly different from the traditional billing system that simply takes units of services, applies the charge, and sends in the claim. Almost every data system is designed for this FFS environment, and vendors will be challenged to make changes to allow the collection of more meaningful data. Even more complex will be the likelihood that every system will need to do double duty. FFS will not go away, and it may be years before the shared-savings model becomes a significant portion of the overall care provided in the market. Data systems will need to be effective and efficient in both worlds.

The data systems can be fully functional and able to capture the data needed to support the clinical and financial needs of the organization; however, two critical elements remain: 1) the data must be in a format that can be retrieved in such a way to support clinical and operation decision-making, and 2) provider and business leaders must actually use those data to further refine operations and monitor quality. Data alone will not make the ACO successful.

Shared risk/shared reward

The recent health reform legislation has determined that the ACO is really a shared-savings model. Any reductions in the cost of caring for a defined population from the historic levels are shared among the payer and the providers.

If an ACO functions much like the patient-centered medical home, at least at the primary care level, then it would follow that primary physicians will likely increase their costs as they add staff to track patients through the system and lose some revenue if they begin to respond to telephone questions rather than bring patients to the office. These costs, in theory, would be offset by bonus dollars derived from the overall reduction in care costs. If specialists continue to order unneeded imaging studies and inpatient episodes are not managed well, then those savings will evaporate and the ACO will likely fail as primary physicians learn they cannot afford to participate. In this example, risk and reward are shared, and that is the foundational theory behind the ACO and a goal that must be addressed during the planning and development process.

What will be common to all is that payers (public or private) and the ACO establish a cost target for the care that they will provide to the enrolled population. It then becomes the responsibility of the ACO to decide who within its provider network gets how much and how those dollars will be paid. This means that shared risk and shared savings exist only within the ACO and not between the provider and the payer.

The HMO model has always had risk pools, which were typically tied to sectors of care and not to the total care provided. PCPs might have some risk/reward tied to referrals to specialists and specialists to diagnostics and admissions, but few would hold the primary physicians accountable for the actions of the surgeon. That changes in the ACO. The primary physician can benefit from or lose revenue from the surgical length of stay, as can the hospital.

Many commercial payers have per diem relationships with hospitals; so, within some limits, the hospital will be paid a fixed amount for each day of care. If a patient leaves quickly, the hospital gets paid less (there are typically some benefits and penalties, but these differ widely). Medicare, of course, uses DRGs as the basis of hospital reimbursement, with adjustments based on severity and other factors. This too would change in the ACO. If physicians, ancillary providers, and hospital clinical staff can create an efficient and appropriate care continuum, the patient will either avoid admission or spend the minimum appropriate time in the hospital. That lower cost will translate to a pool of funds that can be shared with the ACO provider network. (More on that topic is addressed in the next chapter.)

At some point, the ACO will need to use financial penalties as a means of behavior modification. Physicians or groups that do not effectively follow treatment protocols will need to receive reduced payments related to the excess care. Hospitals that cannot streamline discharge functions or that do a poor job of case management may see episodes or days that are unreimbursed. It is unlikely that ACOs will have an "everyone wins" or "everyone loses" model of payment. This will add a level of complexity that makes the ACO even more of a challenging undertaking.

Summary

Although the ultimate model of an ACO may differ by market and sponsor, all will share a common feature. They will be complex organizations delivering an unproven product. The learning curve for providers will be steep, the infrastructure needed to support the operations of the ACO will be complex, and the member-patients may be hesitant or resistive. Ultimately, the patient will need to believe that the care they receive is as good or better than in the past, that it is delivered in a way that is not overly restrictive (Americans do not like long waits and rules), and financial incentives are provided for tolerating the changes. A lot can be learned from the gatekeeper HMO model of the 1980s; it is important to take the time to educate the patient about why certain care policies are in place and expend the effort to make the patient a partner in his or her care. The least expensive disease to treat is the one that is avoided.

REFERENCES

1. Regional Variation in Medicare Service Use, Report to the Congress, January 2011. Medicare Payment Advisory Commission. *www.medpac.gov/documents/Jan11_RegionalVariation_report.pdf.* Accessed January 11, 2011.

2. "Health, United States, 2010." *www.cdc.gov/nchs/hus.htm.* Accessed February 16, 2011.

Physician-Hospital Integration

Integration among physicians and hospitals is occurring at a record pace. A previous wave of integration, which generally denoted employment of physicians by hospitals, started in the 1990s and, to some extent, reached an apex in the middle to latter part of that decade. However, it was not long until many health systems divested their employed physician groups—a trend that transpired over several years. Then history repeated itself, as it often does, when a whole new dynamic of integration began to emerge in the first decade of the 21st century. Although many of the structures were similar to what occurred in the '90s, a new term—*alignment*—surfaced that describes the current affiliations between hospitals and physicians more accurately. Alignment is a broader term than employment; one of the primary drivers of alignment is the prospect of changes in reimbursement paradigms, first by the government and later by the private payers. Thus, alignment strategies in recent years largely resulted from anticipated and/or realized changes in reimbursement and reimbursement structures.

ACOs as a Driver of Alignment

In the strictest sense, alignment can occur among fellow providers (i.e., private practices to private practices); more likely, alignment is in the context of physicians and hospitals/health systems. Many physicians and hospitals find that joining hospital consortiums offers the benefits they seek, and the consortiums appear to be the best response to changes in reimbursement.

Many specialties and testing procedures have undergone reductions in reimbursement. In 2008, Medicare began making unprecedented cuts in diagnostic testing reimbursement for cardiology, long before accountable care organizations (ACO) appeared on the reimbursement horizon and prior to the Patient Protection and Affordable Care Act (PPACA) passed in 2010.[1] Such changes have driven physicians to align with hospitals because, for the most part, hospitals have not experienced reimbursement reductions when they bill either within their inpatient facility or on an outpatient prospective payment system basis.

Nonetheless, ACOs will continue to drive integration/alignment and could ultimately result in the two major providers of healthcare (i.e., hospitals and physicians) virtually becoming one from a provider delivery/reimbursement standpoint. This means that the government and other payers may only recognize one provider in terms of issuing reimbursement for services, and that one provider (i.e., hospitals and physicians) must be aligned fully to receive that reimbursement. Thus, ACOs and physician-hospital alignment are very much a part of the overall equation of understanding how ACOs will work and function in the new healthcare delivery system.

This chapter presents the various alignment models and related considerations that play a major part of the strategies for hospitals and physicians preparing for ACOs, bundled reimbursement, and other changes in the reimbursement system.

Reasons for alignment

Before specifically considering the alignment models, it is imperative to understand the key drivers for alignment, such as the following:

- Declining physician incomes

- Changing physician demographics (many physicians prefer to work fewer hours with more predictable income)

- Probable physician shortages

- Increasing receptivity to full alignment (defined later in this chapter)

- Marginal success in limited forms of alignment

- Opportunity to improve reimbursement

- Stabilizing provider recruitment and retention

- Realizing greater economy of scale in expense and asset purchases, including supplies, technology, and other items

- Reducing physician hassle to manage their practices by malpractice insurance, etc.

- Responding to the changing reimbursement paradigm via ACOs and related structures

These factors are all viable reasons why physicians and hospitals are aligning at a rapid pace. As the government takes the lead in changing the reimbursement paradigm, there are many other environmental and cultural reasons for physicians and hospitals to integrate. The economic factors, coupled with other issues important to physicians, such as quality of life and a lack of desire to own their own business, seem to be aligned for further integration.

Alignment challenges

Alignment has its challenges based on the inherent differences between hospitals and physicians. Primarily, the challenges center on the following perspectives:

- Cultural

- Operational

- Autonomy and control

- Trust

- Competition

- Sharing revenue

These basic differences create challenges with alignment.

Cultural

Hospitals and physicians have very different cultures. Both focus heavily on quality patient care and clinical outcomes, yet their approach is from different perspectives. Hospitals have a high level of bureaucracy, work through multiple tiers of management, and generally employ hundreds of associates. Medical practices are streamlined in their decision-making, can respond more rapidly, and have fewer employees.

Operational

Operationally, hospitals tend to work on a department-by-department basis (almost separately) with some continuity, though separation by service line is quite common. Physician groups (even multispecialty groups) are apt to work collegially and are somewhat dependent on each other for survival.

Autonomy and control

Loss of physician ownership (especially when the physicians are accustomed to autonomy and control) is a major hurdle to overcome. Even physicians who desire less responsibility for the day-to-day practice management prefer some level of control and decision-making over their practices. Although physicians usually maintain control over decision-making in clinical areas when in alignment with hospitals, day-to-day business and administrative decisions are often assumed by the hospital. Governance and leadership issues are a major challenge within alignment structures and often require as much attention as negotiation of the economic terms prior to an affiliation transaction.

Trust

Lack of trust is another major challenge in alignment between hospitals and physicians. Historically, many hospitals and physicians have had a fairly high level of mistrust, although they work together. Without a measure of good faith, it is difficult for any parties to work together, particularly when added to basic cultural differences. Every effort must be made to establish trust between the two parties prior to an affiliation transaction. Even with a solid economic foundation, lack of trust will often impede the success of an affiliation or partnership.

Competition

In many instances, hospitals and physicians have served partially as competitors. Many physicians have developed their own ancillary services, such as ambulatory surgery centers, diagnostic catheterization laboratories, imaging centers, etc., in direct competition to hospitals. Once the affiliation transpires, both parties must "bury the hatchet." They must transition from a competitive to a partnering environment.

Sharing revenue

Another challenge to alignment is sharing of revenue, especially in the ACO environment. Under ACOs, Medicare will continue to reimburse providers under their current agreement (fee-for-service [FFS] payments, diagnosis-related groups [DRG], etc.) according to the final regulations. If a Centers for Medicare & Medicaid Services (CMS) ACO entity successfully meets all quality and financial goals, the ACO will be awarded a savings amount which is to be "shared" among all ACO participants. How the new savings revenue is shared between providers is determined by the ACO during the set-up of the legal entity. The sharing algorithm could be a great challenge for the ACO participants to establish due to the dynamics of the core goals of an ACO: reduced hospitalizations, reduced ER visits, improved quality, etc. Clearly, the greater healthcare dollars are incurred with inpatient admissions; it must be the focus of the primary care physicians (PCP) and specialists to work together to manage chronic and acute conditions to avoid hospitalizations while still ensuring quality patient care. So, physicians work diligently to reduce admissions, hospitals receive less reimbursement dollars due to fewer acute and ER admissions, the ACO achieves savings (and meets the quality goals)—and how will these savings be shared equitably across all provider participants? In many instances, the hospitals may not have participated in the care of some patients, yet they would be eligible to share in the savings based upon the provisions of their ACO. Although this could create some internal challenges with the participating healthcare providers, the overall recognition of a well-managed patient fits the goals and objectives of the ACO structure. As such, the sharing among all providers is both reasonable and fair.

Different Alignment Models

Alignment and integration arrangements take various shapes and forms, usually in three major models: limited alignment models, moderate alignment models, and full alignment models. How these various models will be affected by ACOs is still unclear. As private ACO requirements are defined fully, hospitals and physicians will have to explore their alignment options. Private ACOs that existed in 2010, 2011, and into 2012 offered different alignment options for hospitals and physicians. Some physician-only ACOs were created to focus on patients (not necessarily Medicare beneficiaries) with chronic conditions such as diabetes and heart disease. However, the majority of the private ACOs include hospitals and physicians.

Limited alignment arrangements

Limited alignment arrangements can encompass managed care networks, call-coverage stipends, medical directorships, and recruitment guarantees. The discussions that follow relate to the role these limited alignment arrangements will play in forming ACOs.

Managed care networks

Managed care networks are a basic form of limited alignment, usually established through independent practice associations (IPA) and/or physician-hospital organizations (PHO). Many have been in operation for a number of years and have definite benefit. Interestingly, as hospitals and physicians begin to form ACOs, many hospitals are reassessing their PHOs and considering them as viable foundations for meeting ACO standards. PHOs have been loosely formed alliances among fellow providers. Although they represent minimal integration, and fall far short of merging hospitals and physicians or fellow physicians, they have the potential to serve as the basis for forming an ACO.

Historically, IPAs and PHOs are created to allow their members to jointly contract for reimbursement. Recently, the Federal Trade Commission (FTC) has challenged these structures relative to potential antitrust violations. Essentially, PHOs and IPAs negotiate FFS contracts without meeting legal requirements for clinical integration. Clinical integration allows a PHO to negotiate FFS contracts. The clinical integration question will have to be addressed under ACOs. Originally, when IPAs and PHOs were negotiating capitated contracts, this form of financial integration did not require clinical integration. ACOs will require clinical integration in order to meet the patient-centered, quality, and cost reduction goals. A CMS ACO will not negotiate contracts with Medicare because each participating provider will continue to receive the current contracted reimbursement as a free-standing hospital, physician, or other healthcare provider. However, it is safe to say that PHOs and IPAs will have a role in alignment models whether within or outside of any type of ACO.

Call-coverage stipends

Pay-for-call is a popular form of compensation for physicians that serve in the hospital's emergency department (ED) call rotation and are directed to unassigned patients who present in the ED. Previously, physicians performed call coverage without pay, as the service served as a source of new patients. Further, the physician was able to bill for the professional fees for services rendered in the hospital ED. Unfortunately, as payer mix challenges have increased, the number of paying patients that appear in the ED has diminished dramatically. The average ED patient is often uninsured, self-paying, or nonpaying. Therefore, physicians that take calls without pay sacrifice their time and income on many levels.

Hospitals are bound to provide care for all individuals who appear in their ED because of the federal Emergency Medical Treatment and Labor Act (EMTALA). Also known as the Consolidated Omnibus Budget Reconciliation Act of 1985 or the patient antidumping law, EMTALA requires hospitals to provide an examination and treatment to stabilize the patient without any consideration of that patient's ability to pay—whether they have insurance or not. Physicians not bound by EMTALA, however, are less willing to provide patient care without some compensation. For these reasons, more physicians are receiving remuneration from hospitals for being on call.

The ways to compensate physicians on call vary, even for employed physicians (who are thus fully aligned with the hospital). The key point is whether the pay-for-call arrangement for physicians qualifies as sufficient alignment with a hospital for being a part of an ACO. As a very limited form of alignment, pay-for-call alignment does not provide enough integration between the hospital and the physician to even come close to being a part of an ACO setting. An exception would be for those physicians already employed or fully aligned with a hospital who have negotiated pay-for-call as an additional component of their compensation. Although not directly related to ACO involvement, this would be a part of the overall integration with the hospital, with employment being the key point that allows them to be a part of an ACO.

Medical directorships

Medical directorships are a long-standing but limited form of integration between physicians and hospitals. In these arrangements, the physician is contracted through a professional services agreement (PSA) to provide clinical oversight over a particular department, service line, or other operation within the hospital. The physician is compensated at fair market value, which allows the hospital to maintain a needed service and provides limited alignment between the hospital and the physicians.

Medical directorships alone do not serve as an alignment model that will promote ACOs, and they do not provide a vehicle for developing an ACO. Nevertheless, as ACOs form and mature, particularly those that grow large and cover a wide spectrum of services, medical directorships could provide clinical oversight regarding the overall ACO functions.

Recruitment guarantees

Hospitals historically have given aid to physicians in private practice through recruitment assistance. The Stark Law's exception for physician recruitment arrangements allows this action when hospitals can justify both a community need and benefit from the physician specialty recruited. Although this process is subject to substantial regulatory scrutiny, it has traditionally been a major, though limited, form of alignment. Because the recruited physician enters private practice, he or she is not directly integrated (at least long-term) with the hospital. Moreover, that physician is not obligated to work with that hospital. Further, the recruitment guarantee loan is forgiven entirely as long as the physician continues to work in the service area, not in any particular hospital.[2]

Another form of alignment is an incubation model wherein the hospital employs the physician for a limited period and then places him or her in the private practice. After that limited period, usually one to three years, the physician moves into the private practice, without full alignment or integration with the hospital.

Although recruitment incentives (including incubation arrangements) are a viable alignment strategy, they do not provide any significant support in the context of ACOs. Moreover, the recruited physician under hospital support would best be a hospital employee to link to an ACO.

Moderate alignment initiatives

Moderate forms of alignment encompass management services organizations (MSO), targeted cost incentives, joint ventures, and clinical co-management/service line management. This section describes each of these initiatives in relation to ACOs.

Management services organizations

MSOs are entities that can be created by both hospitals and physicians (or joint ventures) to provide a myriad of services to their "client" practices and other healthcare entities. MSOs can offer group purchasing as well as services. With the current heavy emphasis in healthcare on information technology (IT), information services organizations (ISO) are often the focus of MSOs.

MSOs are a viable moderate-level alignment strategy. MSOs and ISOs may well be a part of the ACO continuum as they emerge on the healthcare scene. MSOs could form a part of the ACO in its overall structure and complexion.

Hypothetically, a practice that is seasoned and sophisticated in its healthcare delivery models may well be able to spin off an MSO-ISO. This entity could serve as the platform or foundation for providing a cross-section of group purchasing (e.g., supplies, IT, malpractice insurance, etc.), plus specific management services from revenue cycle/billing and collections to total management of the client practice or other healthcare entity. In this sense, the MSO-ISO could become a significant link in consolidating a large field of healthcare providers ultimately to form an ACO.

KEY COMPONENTS OF MSOs/ISOs

As the regulations are published and ACOs are better defined, the role of management services organizations may well be a significant part of the full continuum. The following are key elements of MSOs/ISOs.

- Management support services through MSOs is a viable way for hospitals to be involved in medical practice management and marketing support services.

- A typical MSO can feature myriad competencies. For example, hospital management support services could encompass the following:

  - Brokering services wherein hospitals refer physicians to an approved list of consultants or service entities

  - In-house hospital medical practice recruitment services

  - In-house hospital medical practice consultants

  - Hospital-based billing/collection services and revenue cycle management services

  - Joint ventures with outside revenue cycle management companies and consultants forming the MSO

  - Hospital-owned comprehensive medical practice management and marketing services

- Historically, independent practices have resisted hospital initiatives in these areas, taking the point of view that it is an unwelcomed intrusion into their own private business affairs.

- This has been responded to in many instances by forming affiliations with outside practice management firms/consultants or forming joint equity MSOs wherein physicians are partners.

The Healthcare Executive's Guide to ACO Strategy

KEY COMPONENTS OF MSOs/ISOs (CONT.)

- MSOs can also be accomplished through the offering of IT. This could be a major level of competency that future MSOs provide, especially with the government mandates for the development of advanced technology within practices, including electronic health records.

- With the incentives that are being provided in such areas, hospitals may be able to provide up to 85% of the cost of the technology. (**Note:** Before committing to making such a huge investment in developing an MSO, completion of a medical staff survey is highly recommended, to assess the true level of interest in subscribing to these services.)

- Before making a large investment in an ACO.

- MSO core competencies:

  - Business development

    - Practice audit process

    - Market plan development

    - Patient acquisition strategies

    - Patient retention strategies

    - Managed care contracting

    - Physician feedback system

The Healthcare Executive's Guide to ACO Strategy

KEY COMPONENTS OF MSOs/ISOs (CONT.)

- Human resources

  - Training programs

  - Performance evaluation

  - Interviewing

  - Job bid system

  - Compensation design

- Accounting

  - Financial statements/bookkeeping

  - Payroll

  - Accounts payable management

  - Expense management

  - Accounts receivable management

- Operations

  - Scheduling

  - Registration

  - Insurance verification

  - Medical records

KEY COMPONENTS OF MSOs/ISOs (CONT.)

- Telephone

- Supplies

- Facility management

– Physician recruitment

  - Internal database development

  - Target marketing

  - Physician compensation/support packages

  - Recruitment firm profiles

  - Contracting

– Physician reimbursement/Revenue cycle management

  - Charge capture

  - Claims processing

  - Follow-up (third party)

  - Collections (self-pay)

  - Cash application

  - Adjustments

  - Denials/appeals

KEY COMPONENTS OF MSOs/ISOs (CONT.)

- - Fee analysis

- - Regulatory issues

- - Enrollee verification

- Information technology

  - - Operating procedures

  - - Backup/recovery procedures

  - - Help desk/problem resolution

  - - Integrated telephone and data network

  - - User manuals and procedures

  - - Communication methodology

  - - Application and technology maintenance and upgrade

  - - System scheduling

- Contracting

  - - Fee service negotiating

  - - Capitation

  - - Communication to offices

  - - Contract renewal

KEY COMPONENTS OF MSOs/ISOs (CONT.)
- Marketing plan
- Open enrollment
– Patient management
- Orientation letter/brochure
- Patient history
- Telephone follow-up
- Patient compliance/monitoring
- Treatment protocols
- Resource usage/norms
- Quality assurance indicators
- Patient satisfaction survey

Source: Coker Group, Advanced IPA Contracting, 2008.

Targeted cost incentives

Targeted cost incentives are a major part of the goals of ACOs to control the spiraling U.S. healthcare costs. Controlling cost is no longer an option: it is mandatory to control expenses and reduce the overall cost of delivery in both absolute dollars as well as cost per procedure, cost per patient, etc. One of the ways to accomplish this is through sharing of additional reimbursement because of realizing such savings.

Relative to hospitals and physicians and alignment, the concept of sharing cost savings has been referred to as gainsharing. Receptivity to gainsharing arrangements has fluctuated and has at times been challenged from a viewpoint of regulatory compliance. In the prospective ACO concept of integration and targeted cost savings, this concept centers more on the savings realized on an overall basis, which in turn would result in greater reimbursement from Medicare through the ACO structure. From an alignment or physician-hospital integration standpoint, the two would share this savings within the ACO and distribute it to its participating members (i.e., physicians and hospitals).

Quality and quality outcomes are other facets of this concept, which are closely aligned with patient satisfaction. ACOs will place a great deal of emphasis on these factors within their proposed structure and makeup. The government will pay ACOs that can demonstrate cost savings, as well as improved quality and patient satisfaction outcomes. The government has a recent history of paying for performance and measured quality through its Physician Quality and Reporting System (PQRS; formerly the Physician Quality Reporting Initiative) program. Since their onset in recent years, many practices have taken advantage of additional reimbursements Medicare has paid as a result of specifically demonstrating compliance with certain quality metrics/indicators. These programs are classified by major specialty service; although they have not yielded significant additional reimbursement, the programs have increased the overall receipts from Medicare versus what they would otherwise have been. (**Note:** The PQRS is a part of the Medicare reimbursement system that is in effect a precursor of pay-for-quality performance. For more information concerning this system, refer to *www.cms. gov/PQRS*.)

Thus, the forms of alignment related to targeted cost savings, quality outcomes, and additional reimbursement are a significant component of the ACO reimbursement paradigm. As an alignment strategy, though moderate forms of integration or alignment, they are an important part of the process.

Many hospitals are already pursuing these concepts by employing physicians or aligning with them, often through PSAs. Here, a portion of the physician's compensation is tied to performance and cost savings. Some more progressive health systems and private groups are preparing for ACOs in this manner, even if they have not yet formed an ACO.

Joint ventures

Joint ventures are a major consideration within the overall alignment strategy and can be structured to accommodate several different endeavors. They take on various roles, structures, and formations within the overall healthcare delivery provider system, such as MSOs/ISOs, as discussed previously. In addition, joint venture arrangements can focus on specialty hospitals, freestanding centers, and other consortiums that provide healthcare delivery.

Block leases are also a part of the joint venture processes. Block leases are agreements where the lessee (usually physician surgeons) agrees to rent the facility (e.g., operating room within an ambulatory surgery center) and often staff and other support systems in total for a defined period. During that period, the lessee has virtually complete control over the facility, analogous to any other lease. The lease is usually for a defined "block" of time each day/week/month.

Joint ventures are subject to many regulations: Stark and anti-kickback legislation, Internal Revenue Service guidelines, tax exempt status, and state regulations, in particular. Although viable as an alignment strategy, they require tremendous scrutiny, planning, and attention to matters of compliance.

As of October 1, 2009, "under arrangement" joint ventures ceased to be legal entities. Therefore, joint venture arrangements must be vetted to ensure risks of noncompliance. Even certain fully aligned models like PSAs (see the following discussion) must be carefully crafted to avoid any "under arrangement" characteristics.

As relates to ACOs, it is doubtful that specific joint ventures would be applicable other than within the context of being the beginning of the continuum of alignment that ultimately would allow for an ACO to be formed from within the joint venture entity (but not in and of itself the joint venture). Although this may be inconsistent with what we discussed regarding MSOs, it really is not that MSOs may in fact form the foundation for the actual ACO entity. To that extent, if it is a joint venture MSO, it would qualify to be a part of the ACO-formed entity. Nonetheless, most joint ventures would not qualify as a source ultimately to become an ACO. However, the CMS regulations do allow joint ventures to participate in an ACO, providing they follow all legal requirements of a CMS ACO.

Clinical co-management/service line management

Similar limited forms of alignment structures, but with some differences, are clinical co-management and service line management agreements.

Clinical co-management entails specific clinical protocols and structures within a particular service line (e.g., neurosurgery, general surgery, orthopedics, cardiology, etc.). Both operational and quality targets are established that enhance the overall coordination and continuum of care plus strive for improved quality while controlling cost. Although these arrangements have the key components to qualify for ACOs, they stop short of forming an ACO.

Essentially, service line management encompasses all services that the physicians would provide within a particular specialty within the hospital, even to the point of helping to assist in the management processes. Some previous forms of alignment, such as call, could be a part of the service line agreement in that the physicians might be providing call as a part of the service line agreement.

Service line management also may be a part of the overall alignment strategy. These arrangements either can be distinctive or they can be a part of a co-management agreement. Service line and clinical co-management agreements serve to further align hospitals and physicians, stopping short of full alignment, or they can be a part of the full alignment strategy. Often called "wraparound" agreements, essentially they are in addition to the basic form of full alignment, which may be employment or by PSA. In effect, these agreements—whether co-management or service line management—are PSAs, but here they are distinguished from the global payment PSA and/or other extensive forms of alignment as discussed subsequently.

Clinical co-management and service line management, as discussed, offer some features that would complement ACO formation; yet, they are not sufficient to justify a foundation for an ACO.

Full alignment arrangements

Highly integrated models include three major components, all of which look like or are significantly similar to employment. The following section on full alignment addresses the clinic model, employment model, and PSAs for comprehensive professional services.

Clinic model

The clinic model is a highly integrated health system wherein both the clinic and the hospitals are fully aligned—an almost totally seamless operation. In the strictest sense, the clinic model, typified by major clinics such as Mayo Clinic and Cleveland Clinic, regards hospitals as somewhat of an ancillary service. In these types of organizations, physicians are employed by the clinic and have equity in the clinic, which includes all services (e.g., hospital, clinics, diagnostics).

The clinic model is only available for large institutions, such as those named previously. They undoubtedly have the best opportunity or potential for forming ACOs, and in effect are a virtual ACO even before the entity is created. They have the full continuum of services that ACOs will have to provide, encompassing the physician component, hospital component, diagnostics and ancillaries, and other related services in a seamless operation. If private ACOs ultimately provide a bundled payment, the clinic model offers the best structure for delivery of care.

Employment model

Employment can take on many forms and structures that allow full alignment between physicians and hospitals.

Physician employment can be structured in a number of ways, but typically the relationship can be simply described as a "W-2" relationship between the physician and the hospital. This offers the opportunities for complete integration wherein the hospital and physicians are one entity. Hospitals may create subsidiary entities, even for-profit subsidiaries, within nonprofit hospital systems. Basic employment agreements can have many variations. For example, the physicians may be employed by the hospital and yet continue to own and operate their administrative structure through a jointly owned MSO, or the physicians in and of themselves own that entity. In this event, the hospital will pay the physician-owned management entity a management fee at an appropriate fair market value rate. Although a possible arrangement, this model is unusual and rare.

Employment is the most likely scenario for many physicians and hospitals in preparation to meet ACO requirements. Moving quickly toward physician employment, hospitals believe it is the most simple and effective way to prepare for the consolidation of healthcare providers to respond to the proposed reimbursement methodology.

PSA for comprehensive professional services

The final integration model that entails full alignment is the PSA. The PSA is like employment in many ways in that the physicians are completely contracted for services by the hospital. PSAs can also have hybrids of their basic structures. Following are two examples:

- In the first structure, physicians have contracts for professional services, while the hospital employs the physician's staff and owns and manages the administrative structure of the practice.

- In the second PSA structure, sometimes called a *global payment PSA*, the practice is contracted for professional services and continues to control and have the responsibility for all overhead within the arrangement. Overhead encompasses employee benefits and other costs; the practice receives a "top-line" payment from the hospital for professional services.

The pros and cons of these PSA alignment structures are not discussed in this context; the interest is in how they might be responsive to ACOs. In these examples, physicians are fully aligned/integrated with the hospital. Therefore, these PSA models, however varied, are viable ACO platforms.

Summary of alignment models

Many physicians perceive that hospitals have deep pockets and can afford virtually any amount (within regulatory parameters of fair market value and commercially reasonable amounts). They believe, therefore, that they will realize their prior levels of income through alignment. This may not be the case and is unlikely under an ACO. As the revenue pie shrinks, the stresses that are on physician groups are being offloaded to hospitals. The question of how long hospitals will be able to absorb such transfers of economic responsibility is clearly unknown. As ACOs become more prominent, presumably transcending the private/commercial sector, this dynamic could become a greater challenge.

Discussion of various alignment models in this chapter has focused on how initiatives may best respond to an ACO structure along with their overall reimbursement characteristics. Figure 4.1 summarizes what might result.

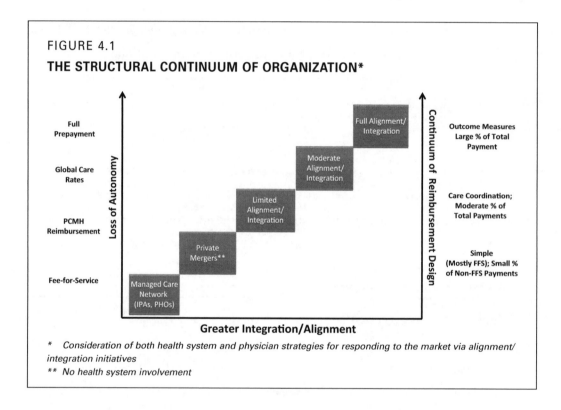

FIGURE 4.1

THE STRUCTURAL CONTINUUM OF ORGANIZATION*

*   Consideration of both health system and physician strategies for responding to the market via alignment/integration initiatives
** No health system involvement

The intent of this figure is for hospitals and physicians to develop an informed strategy for physician/hospital integration in the context of this new reimbursement paradigm. Fully integrated delivery systems are much more feasible going forward in order to ensure the receipt of the full potential payment that will be offered to the ACO, and that is done with greater coordination of care and process structure, for example. The feasibility increases as these strategies move from small practices and unrelated hospitals to IPAs/PHOs, then on to fully integrated delivery systems among hospitals and physicians.

Continuum of Care and Physician-Hospital Integration

Physicians and hospital executives often ask how ACOs will affect their practices and their working relationships. With CMS publishing the final regulations, it appears that PPACA requirements for physicians and hospitals to work together will increase. Several major factors are likely to occur from the onset. They include the following:

- From an organizational structure, the patient-centered medical home (PCMH) and the ACO are likely structures that will develop and be required.

- From a payment reform standpoint, a system will evolve where outcomes payments and bundled payments will become the more common or the total form of reimbursement. Under any circumstances wherein these new organizational structures and new forms of payment become the standard, physicians and hospitals must be aligned. Therefore, answers to the question of physicians and hospital executives are in the context of these two dramatically new structures. Although the final CMS regulations do not included bundled payments, it is likely that such reimbursement models could be included in revised provisions for the second CMS ACO contract periods beginning in 2016. Additionally, some private ACOs may use bundled payments or capitation in their reimbursement models. It should be noted that in August 2011, the CMS Innovation Center launched the *Bundled Payments for Care Improvement Initiative*. This initial program has four models available for participation by healthcare providers. CMS plans to use the results of this program to determine future initiatives.

The ACO structure may have several PCMH entities that will contract with the ACO via independent physicians. In addition, PCMH entities can originate from a hospital-employed multispecialty group environment. In this case, the two parties (i.e., the independent physicians that are contracted along with the health system employed multispecialty group) would form a clinically integrated network that would ultimately become a part of the ACO. As previously discussed, the ACO would be best formed through various integration models. Ideally, it would also be easiest formed through some existing relationship such as full alignment (e.g., employment, PSA, or lesser forms of alignment such as a PHO/IPA/MSO scenario). Thus, within the integration concept, ACOs will continue to be provider-led organizations whose mission is to oversee and manage a full continuum of care to be accountable for both quality outcomes and costs associated with the provision of those services. All of this would be performed within a defined population group. Physician-hospital integration, therefore, is essential for achieving optimum levels of this continuum of care that will help attain cost control and improve quality.

Integration between hospitals and physicians is imperative to provide this full continuum of care. As presented previously, there are multiple forms of ACOs, such as:

- Fully-integrated delivery system between hospitals and physicians where the physicians are employed (or virtually employed) through a PSA

- PHOs and IPAs where the connection emanates from such entities

- Multispecialty group practices (with or without hospital ownership), possibly with corresponding adjunct MSOs

- Independent networks of physician practices, which include hospital-employed physicians and both independent and specialty PCPs, though in all likelihood this latter entity must have some legal structure that ties all of these entities together

The key to continuum of care is achieving clinical integration among these entities. By definition, *clinical integration* is "an active and ongoing program to evaluate and modify practice patterns by the network's physician participants and create a high degree of interdependence and cooperation among the physicians to control costs and ensure quality."[3]

This program may include the following three factors:

1. Establishing mechanisms to monitor and control use of healthcare services that are designed to control costs and assure quality of care

2. Selectively choosing network physicians who are likely to further these efficiency objectives

3. Significantly investing in capital—both monetary and human—
    in the necessary infrastructure and capability to realize the
    claimed efficiencies

In the definition of 15 years ago, the FTC and Department of Justice were looking
for clinical integration to address the development and maturation of clinical
protocols that hopefully would dictate higher levels of quality and lower costs.
They were also looking for a continuum of care review based on the application
of those protocols. Next, they were considering tools that would ensure physician
compliance to those protocols. Finally, the "tie that binds" for all of this to work
was a common IT system to ensure that patient data relevant to the continuum of
care was achieved.

Although this was some 15 years ago and little has been done in that period to
achieve these goals and the overall continuity/continuum of care, the ACO concept and related physician-hospital integration requirements will bring this to a
new level of maturity. At the core of physician-hospital integration and achieving
high levels of continuum of care is a clinically integrated network. Physicians
and hospitals must be linked more than ever before. Models in this chapter are
merely means to an end to achieve the goal of clinical integration. Achieving these
lofty goals calls for significant planning and "deal-making" between physicians
and hospitals.

An organized delivery system is a consortium of organizations that work together
to provide an organized continuum of services to a specified population. That
organized group (hospitals and physicians for the most part) must be willing to be

held both fiscally and clinically accountable for the outcomes and overall health of that defined population. In essence, this is a textbook definition of PCMH and ACOs. Characteristics of such highly performing integrated delivery systems must include the following:[4]

- Strong physician leadership

- Organizational structure

- Clear shared aims

- Governance

- Accountability and transparency

- Selection and workforce planning

- Patient-centered teams

In order to achieve such a continuum of care, there are many variations that range from less integrated structures to more integrated structures. From the less integrated structure perspective, we typically move from small (even solo) physician practices and groups plus individual hospitals to single-specialty groups and hospital consolidation/affiliation. To further this along, we may include the fully integrated hospital and physician network; from the hospital's perspective, some academic faculty practices may be included.

The more integrated systems at the beginning include a multispecialty group that is already affiliated with hospitals, then moving this into a truly integrated delivery system such as the Mayo Clinic, Ochsner Health System, and others. Within the final continuum of a fully integrated system that would also include the payer perspective, the final goal would be a Kaiser Permanente, for example.

Wherever a hospital or physician group is at this point, the ultimate goal is somewhere down the continuum of achieving an integrated structure. Various forms of physician-hospital alignment, discussed in this chapter, are step stones along the path. For example, service line management, a moderate form of integration, is a good starting point to joint accountability and management—or dyadic management—of an entire hospital service line, which theoretically should go a long way toward achieving improved quality and contained costs. When hospitals and physicians are motivated through financial integration to be at the table on a regular basis, discussing how they can achieve better quality and cost measures/goals and targets, it undoubtedly will improve overall performance. This is at the core of ACOs' goals and objectives and the overall patient-focused continuum of care concepts throughout this book and in this chapter.

Structures between hospitals and physicians can move into more direct partnerships beyond service lines into clinical operation leadership teams and to the executive level of hospitals and/or physician groups. The overarching goal is to achieve a better product (or result) than is currently being achieved, with comparable or better quality, at lower cost.

The achievement of more acceptable clinical and financial outcomes requires significant forethought, planning, and implementation, even after the physician-hospital integration models have been undertaken. There are important operational and workflow principles that must be part of any physician-hospital integration model that ultimately may become a part of an ACO and its overall goals and objectives.

For example, from an operational standpoint, actions relative to the ACO should improve the credibility (and reliability) of operational flows that are consistent and proven to be effective in their approach. An electronic health record (EHR) system must be the primary vehicle or tool to develop such consistencies; yet an EHR is only the vehicle or tool for achieving this—not the ultimate answer.

Workflow principles should be a part of the planning process for the assurance of continuum of care. Consideration of workflow principles includes:

- Elimination of non–value-added functions

- Continued automation of work that should be done outside of the actual physician/patient encounter

- Delegation of work that could be done by nonprovider staff, when possible (at lower cost)

- Tools that trigger reminders to the providers of things that must occur before the patient leaves that ensure higher levels of efficiency in care

- Shifting some of the responsibilities through EHR and other matters to the patient to offload some of the cost of care

When these actions become a part of the ACO and are ingrained into the physician-hospital integration model, the ACO will be able to demonstrate lower cost and higher quality.

Summary

This chapter has reviewed various possibilities for physician-hospital integration, ranging from very limited to complete alignment. Many physicians are not ready for full alignment and are uninterested at this point. Hospitals, also, are struggling to define where they fit within this continuum. As ACOs become the customary or the required structure to achieve reimbursement, it is essential for every hospital and every physician to plan for integration and alignment with one another. Even limited forms of alignment will be necessary; in time, full alignment may be required for all providers. Time will tell what is required in this context as this new system of payment and reimbursement settles into place and becomes the standard for the future of healthcare delivery.

REFERENCES

1. Public Law 111-148—Mar. 23, 2010 124 Stat. 119. *http://frwebgate.access.gpo.gov/cgi-bin/getdoc. cgi?dbname=111_cong_public_laws&docid=f:publ148.pdf*. Accessed February 24, 2011.

2. Miller, J.B., "Hospital-physician recruitment arrangements," *Physicians News Digest*, May 2003. *www.physiciansnews.com/law/503miller.html*. Accessed February 25, 2011.

3. Department of Justice and Federal Trade Commission Statements of Antitrust Enforcement in Healthcare. 1996.

4. Anthony Shih, Karen Davis, Stephen C. Schoenbaum, Anne Gauthier, Rachel Nuzum, and Douglas McCarthy, Organizing the U.S. Healthcare Delivery System for High Performance, The Commonwealth Fund, August 2008.

5

Compensation and Anticipated Changes

One of the key concerns regarding the onset of accountable care organizations (ACO) is the impact they will have on reimbursement structures, physician productivity, and compensation. As it relates to reimbursement, the key question is whether there will be major changes to the fee-for-service (FFS) environment that largely permeates today's current healthcare industry. Several options were reviewed and the Centers for Medicare & Medicaid Services (CMS) have decided to maintain the current FFS reimbursement schedules and add a shared savings program. However, this does not preclude them from changing the program in 2016, when the second contract period is scheduled to begin. In May 2011, CMS announced a new program that was intended to attract well-established groups that have extensive experience in the principles of the goals of an ACO. This new program, the Pioneer ACO Model, will provide accelerated reimbursements to those entities that meet the quality, cost reduction, and patient satisfaction goals. In year three of the Pioneer program, participating ACOs that demonstrated savings during the first two years will be eligible to receive a significant amount of their future reimbursement from a population-based model. In other words, they will move to a capitation reimbursement model, or a per member payment for part of their revenue.

The changing reimbursement model does not only impact actual reimbursement received but can also, directly and indirectly, impact how physician productivity is measured and physicians' actual productivity. Further, with productivity often driving compensation, the changing reimbursement structures can also impact what a physician will be paid for his or her services.

Historical and Current Reimbursement Structures

Historically and currently, the primary payer of healthcare services is the insurance company and not the patient. This is not likely to change in the near future. The first time a sickness clause was inserted into an insurance contract was in 1847; however, health insurance in its primary form really did not come into play until the late 1920s, when Blue Cross first covered teachers in the state of Texas. In 1932, a citywide plan was implemented in Sacramento, CA, but health insurance as an industry did not really gain prominence until after World War II.[1] Of course, Medicare did not come into play until 1965, when the Social Security Act established the Medicare and Medicaid programs.

Insurance companies (including governmental payers) who foot the bill for the majority of healthcare costs have attempted various methods to control healthcare spending due to the impact on profits to for-profit insurance companies; additionally, the government simply cannot sustain its current spending track, especially with the realized impact of baby boomers. These methods have largely focused on restructuring reimbursement to the providers of healthcare services.

The following section explores the following forms of historical and current reimbursement:

- FFS

- Managed care

- High-deductible health plans

- Capitation

- Incentive models

Fee-for-service

The FFS reimbursement process largely dominates the current healthcare industry and takes on various forms in terms of the actual structure of an insurance policy. Fundamentally, the FFS reimbursement process simply means that providers of healthcare services receive a set fee for each unit of service they provide to patients. For example, if a doctor sees a patient for a common cold, based on the services he or she provides and bills (i.e., current procedural terminology code), he or she will receive a set fee from the insurance company for that specific service. The same would be true for a surgical procedure, hospital stay, etc. Thus, the more work performed/services provided, the more reimbursement received. The FFS model is the basis for Medicare and many other commercial payer reimbursements.

Some perceive the FFS model to be one of the (if not the) key problems with healthcare spending because it creates a strong incentive to "do more" as opposed to focusing on quality outcomes. This has led to much discussion concerning the need for the industry to move from FFS to fee-for-value. This problem is unique to healthcare because other industries naturally move in the direction of fee-for-value, because consumers are not willing to pay for something that does not have value, measured in terms of quality, satisfaction, cost, etc. Because the recipients of services (patients) are not the primary payers of the services (the insurance companies), this natural progression does not exist on an overarching level. Thus, to providers, an FFS approach to reimbursement results in low risk and limited accountability in terms of quality, outcomes, satisfaction, etc.

Managed care

Managed care plans are another common form of reimbursement and are based on contractual agreements between an insurance company and various providers of healthcare services (physicians, hospitals, ancillary services, and others) in order to offer services to a defined population of insured patients. These plans use a contracted payment schedule that dictates what the various providers will be paid for their services. The intent of these plans is to control the cost of care.[2]

The most common forms of managed care are HMOs, point of service (POS) plans, preferred provider organizations (PPO), and primary care case management programs. These plans have a similar intent in terms of attempting to control the cost of care, but vary in terms of the level of flexibility to the patient. For example, HMOs tend to be the most restrictive, limiting patients' ability to see providers outside the network. Further, the HMO often employs physicians providing services in an HMO. Finally, in this type of arrangement, primary care physicians (PCP) play an important role in coordinating the care of the patient.

Thus, the patient must go through his or her PCP in order to receive care from other specialty providers. PPOs and POS plans tend to be less restrictive in terms of allowing the patients more flexibility in choosing their providers, with the PCP still playing an important role but acting less like a gatekeeper.

High-deductible health plans

In recent years, high-deductible health plans have gained prominence, largely because they are less costly than "traditional" plans from an employer's perspective. These plans still function similarly to managed care/FFS plans from the provider's perspective but are very different from the patient's perspective. These plans shift the initial burden of payment for services to the patient until a certain deductible is met each plan year. For example, the deductible may be $5,000, wherein the patient is responsible for all healthcare costs up to the $5,000 deductible and then all costs thereafter are 100% covered. The intent of these plans is to shift more of the burden of payment to the patient, wherein he or she becomes more cognizant of his or her use of healthcare services, as the out-of-pocket cost is more substantial.

The key difference for providers with these plans is that more of the payment is coming from the patient and not an insurance company. Thus, although the reimbursement ultimately received may be the same, the ability to collect becomes more challenging because collection must occur at the patient level and not at the insurance level. The same difference impacts patients. In a traditional plan, it may only cost a $15 copayment to see a PCP, whereas in a high-deductible health plan the patient may pay the full cost of the visit, perhaps $100. Thus, out-of-pocket costs are more substantial.

Capitation

In the 1980s, as a combatant to the FFS model, capitation arrangements began to see increasing prominence. In capitation arrangements, providers are paid a set fee, often on a per patient basis, for the full management of that group of patients for a set period of time. Thus, there is no payment when services are actually rendered, but the per patient/per period payment covers the full continuum of services for that set period.

Capitation is fundamentally the opposite of FFS in that each time the physician renders services to a patient, it results in a cost to the physician that otherwise would not have been incurred. Thus, the incentive in capitation is to limit or control the amount of services actually rendered to patients in an effort to maximize profitability. From an insurance company's perspective, therefore, capitation allows them to lock in their costs for a set period; from a patient's perspective, it may result in less than adequate treatment, as there is actually a disincentive for the physician to see the patient more, perform additional tests, etc.

For the majority of the country, capitation arrangements came and went, but they are still prevalent in certain regions of the country, such as the West Coast and mainly in California.

Incentive models

While incentive models are still in their infancy, many insurance companies, including Medicare, are attempting to insert these types of models into the current reimbursement process. These can differ for each payer, but a global example that is applicable to any provider willing to participate is Medicare's

Physician Quality Reporting System (formerly PQRI). This program was established in 2006 for implementation in 2007 and essentially provided eligible and participating healthcare providers an incentive on their Medicare reimbursement if they tracked and reported on certain quality metrics established by Medicare. Since its inception, this program has been successful, and more quality measures continue to be added to the program.

Summary of historical and current reimbursement methods

There have been numerous reimbursement methodologies attempted over the past several decades in terms of reimbursing healthcare providers for their services. However, managed care and FFS models continue to be the most dominant forms of reimbursement. This is likely a result of the fact that they are rather "simple" models in that you simply track work performed and pay accordingly. It is very black and white, very objective. Further, and not surprisingly, physicians are partial to the FFS model.

Ian Morrison effectively sums up physicians' perspective on FFS in his *H&HN Weekly* article "Chasing Unicorns: The Future of ACOs." "Doctors love fee-for-service. They just want more fee and less service," he writes. The results of a Harris Interactive survey that asked physicians what they thought about physician incentives as a means to reform the reimbursement system showed that doctors were somewhat satisfied with FFS—the current reimbursement method. But they did not like the amount of payment for the level of effort often involved in providing services, he explains. When it comes to changing the reimbursement system, however, the same surveys showed that physicians don't really like any of the payment reform ideas, such as pay-for-performance, bundled payment, or global episodic payment. For example, only about 16% of physicians would be in favor of accepting bundled payment. "The wonks designing bundled payment have not quite thought through the likely bloody wars in every hospital when a sack of money is dumped on the desk to cover all the costs of a hip or knee replacement: the diagnostic workup, the diagnosis-related group payment, the surgeon's fee, the rehabilitation, and the readmission risk. Fights over who gets what will be reminiscent of the second battle in *Braveheart*," Morrison writes.[3]

Factors such as quality, cost control, and satisfaction/patient experience are much more subjective and take a much more sophisticated process to manage and administer. Many of the new reimbursement structures on the horizon attempt to go down this road, focusing more on the overall value of services provided and not just on the fact that the work was performed.

Proposed Reimbursement Structures

The future method of reimbursement is largely up for debate, with most believing that it will be an amalgamation of reimbursement methodologies, some reminiscent of historical reimbursement schemes and others, completely new. This section outlines what is on the horizon from a reimbursement perspective.

Fee-for-service

Many believe that the FFS process will continue to be the backbone of the reimbursement system going forward, with some caveats. The final CMS ACO regulations confirm the continued use of FFS reimbursements, at least during the first contract period ending December 31, 2015. Complete abandonment of the current system overnight is likely untenable for non-ACO providers. Further, much of the healthcare system outside of reimbursement is largely FFS-based. For example, most hospital-employed physician contracts include productivity-based compensation arrangements that pay the physician based on collections, relative value units, or some other measure of productivity. Thus, there is alignment between the overall reimbursement model and the compensation model applied to these physicians, in terms of its focus on the volume of work performed. Therefore, completely disrupting the FFS reimbursement process completely disrupts many of the compensation arrangements currently in place. Thus, a complete abandonment of FFS is unlikely to occur, at least in the near-term.

As previously mentioned, under the Medicare ACOs, claims will be submitted as usual and reimbursement will be made to providers under their current FFS or DRG reimbursement schedules. Any savings amount will be paid to the tax identification number (TIN) of the ACO.

What is unknown is whether ongoing reimbursement will be reduced to allow for an incentive. What we mean by this is whether Medicare (and potentially other payers) will reduce their current FFS reimbursement rates to push more ACOs towards reliance on incentive payments that come from the cost savings programs, as they will be needed to ensure all costs in the medical practice and/or hospital are covered. Because this process is intended to control costs, the latter seems untenable (i.e., not reducing FFS reimbursement), at least in the long-term. The final CMS regulations clearly state the FFS reimbursement will be made based upon "current" schedules; however, there is always the possibility that those schedules could be amended in the future.

If ongoing reimbursement is reduced, it will be interesting to see how this plays out because it could have significant cash flow ramifications for many healthcare providers. Meaning, if a substantial portion of a payer mix is Medicare and the reimbursement for these patients is modified to where only a portion is received on an ongoing basis, with the remaining paid at a later date only if required metrics are achieved, this will disrupt the ongoing cash that entities have historically received to operate their businesses.

The bottom line is that FFS reimbursement will still play a key role in the reimbursement process for the near future.

Bundled payments

One of the proposed payment reimbursement methodologies that may gain prominence with the onset of ACOs is bundled payments. Some view bundled payments as a payment method that falls between FFS models and capitation arrangements, perhaps allowing for the transition over time. The key concept of this approach is that the providers would assume more financial risk for the cost of services as well as the cost of preventable complications, but not the insurance risk that is involved in capitated arrangements. The key difference is that the physician would not bear the risk of a patient acquiring the condition, as exists with capitation, but would be at risk based on the costs associated with that specific episode of care. Thus, the bundled payment for such services would be based on the average cost of providing this service and therefore providers incurring higher than normal costs would be penalized, with providers who incur lower costs being rewarded. Thus, cost control would be emphasized, as well as coordination among the various providers involved in the service.[4]

The CMS Innovation Center announced the Bundled Payments for Care Improvement Initiative in August 2011. This program was launched as part of the Affordable Care Act and is designed to encourage doctors, hospitals and other healthcare providers to work together to better coordinate care for patients for an episode of care. CMS specifically defines the goals to:

1. Support and encourage providers who are interested in continuously reengineering care to achieve "better health, better care, and lower costs through continuous improvement" (three-part aim outcomes)

2. Create a positively reinforcing cycle that leads to decreasing the cost of an acute episode of care and the associated post-acute care while fostering quality improvement

3. Develop and test payment models that create extended accountability for three-part aim outcomes for acute and post-acute medical care.

4. Shorten the cycle time for adoption of evidence-based care

5. Create environments that stimulate rapid development of new evidence-based knowledge

The bundled payment program proposes three different models, each with different payment protocol. Details regarding the CMS bundled payment program can be found at *http://innovations.cms.gov/initiatives/bundled-payments/index.html*.

The key question with these arrangements is how the bundled payment would be allocated among the various healthcare providers involved in the service. This topic raises significant compliance questions in terms of Stark Law and anti-kickback statutes that largely govern hospital-physician transactions.

One byproduct of concepts such as bundled payments is the somewhat forced alignment between hospitals and physicians. Although not impossible to manage with private practice physicians, the concept of bundled payments would be much easier to accomplish when the physicians providing the services are fully aligned (through employment or another form of alignment) with the hospital. This is because the hospital could simply retain the full bundled payment, paying the physician a fair market wage for his or her professional services.

Medical home payments

The idea of a medical home has been around for several decades but really has not become prevalent in terms of how reimbursement is structured; therefore, the overall concept has not taken off. However, in many instances, the idea of a medical home is synonymous with many of the foundational principles of an ACO. This is because medical homes center on the PCP as the key coordinator of services for patients. In fact, the ACO regulations speak to this synonymy by noting that the regulations preclude duplication in shared savings programs. Meaning, an entity participating as a medical home and receiving shared savings payments cannot also participate in an ACO. Accordingly, we address the specific concept of medical homes in the following, outside of an ACO because we antici-pate many will still occur, at least in the near term.

With this concept, PCPs take on a much greater role in the overall care of a patient because they are not only seeing the patient when the patient presents with a specific ailment but are taking on the task of fully coordinating the care for that patient. This clearly entails additional work that would not be reimbursed under the current FFS model, which is geared toward only compensating for a specific episode of care. Thus, new forms of reimbursement are needed to allow for this concept. Multiple models have been proposed to support this initiative, including one released in January 2011 by the NCQA (National Committee for Quality Assurance), as follows:[5]

- Fee-for-service with adjustments

    - Existing FFS model with new codes for patient-centered medical home efforts

    - Existing FFS model, but with higher payments to account for the full spectrum of services

- Fee-for-service "plus"

    - Existing FFS with lump sum payments to cover the patient-centered medical home work

    - Existing FFS with a per member/per month payment to cover the patient-centered medical home work

- Shared savings model

    - The components of an FFS with adjustments or FFS "plus" model with the inclusion of bonus dollars using one or a combination of the following concepts:

      ○   Pay for performance

      ○   Shared savings

- Comprehensive payment model

    – This would resemble a capitation arrangement, but with some added dollars to encourage the development of the medical home concept; it could also include pay for performance incentives

Capitation

Many believe that capitation will play some role, if not a prominent role, in ACOs in the future. Although not included as part of the Shared Savings Program, CMS does include a per member per month reimbursement under their Pioneer ACO Model. It is possible that some private ACOs may adopt a capitation reimbursement model for their participants.

One difference in this type of capitation versus historical capitation arrangements is that this capitation is at a higher level. Meaning, the capitation arrangement covers both the hospital and multiple physicians in a single contract as opposed to insurance companies entering into separate contracts with the various players. Thus, similar to bundled payments, the ACO concept is forcing closer integration among hospitals and physicians, so that a fully integrated system is likely necessary.[6]

Therefore, the overall idea and concept of capitation is no different from what has been attempted before, only at a higher level. Further, some believe that capitation can be more successful today than in the past due to a variety of factors. These include the fact that many systems are more clinically integrated than during the first wave of integration; information technology and electronic medical records are much more advanced and widespread, leading to better available data; there is more widespread use of clinical guidelines than in previous decades; better risk adjustment methods exist; and there is more experience from past capitation arrangements in terms of what works and does not work.[7]

Blended payment

Blended payments are a key focus of the ACO structure, and many believe that, at least initially, this will likely be the key method of reimbursement for most ACOs. This type of payment was discussed at some length previously in the section on FFS and how FFS reimbursement may change with the onset of ACOs. The CMS Shared Savings program is a blended payment model comprised of the standard FFS reimbursement for physicians and the DRG/FFS for hospitals, with an incentive payment added when quality and cost goals are met.

Many of the private ACOs are using a blended payment model, with carriers reimbursing under their standard fee schedules, and then adding group incentive payments for quality and savings attainment. Some models, primarily those that are physician-only ACOs, use the standard FFS reimbursement model and add an additional payment to PCPs (per patient) for the added time required to coordinate the care across all ACO participants.

Incentive/risk sharing

Incentives and risk sharing will be at the heart of ACOs as a key differentiating factor from the current FFS process where there is no incentive and/or risk other than increases and decreases in use.

At the heart of these incentives is cost control. Meaning, even if an ACO is able to achieve all of the required quality and patient satisfaction, if there is not a minimum reduction in costs, there will be no incentive payment. The ACO regulations require that the pool of potential shared dollars is funded by cost savings and then the amount of payout is based on the quality scoring, up to the maximum amount for each model track. As you will see in Chapter 8, an ACO entity can now remain under Track 1 (the one-sided model) for the entire first contract period. Under Track 1, there is no financial risk sharing for losses. However, the ACO must move to Track 2 for its second and future contract periods, where they will share in both savings and losses.

Medical Home Payment Models

Definite changes are on the horizon relative to reimbursement for medical services. The changes will likely be gradual, with FFS still playing a predominant role early on as the concept of capitation gains more prevalence and becomes engrained in the industry. This expectation is rooted in the fact that some of the proposed reimbursement ideas appear to be transitional methodologies, leading to more capitation-type arrangements, such as the Pioneer ACO Model. Bundled payments clearly give this impression, as does the medical home concept.

Even small changes to the status quo will be a major paradigm shift for all players in the healthcare industry and will require a reevaluation of overall business models, physician compensation arrangements, service offerings, and alignment initiatives. This will clearly be a revolution within the healthcare industry that will likely be in the works for decades. Change does not occur overnight.

Distribution of incentives and allocation of losses

A consideration somewhat ancillary to the previous discussion is how incentives will be distributed. This will play a key role in the overall concept of ACOs. One of the key issues with this topic is securing data to determine how incentives should be distributed. Incentive payments within ACOs will largely be based on quality outcomes, cost control, and patient experience. Each of these components is difficult to track, which means that for incentives to be properly distributed in an ACO, there will need to be complex financial systems to track and report data on a per physician basis, so that when it is time to distribute any incentives, necessary data will be available.

The other key issue in distribution of income involves compliance with Stark Law and anti-kickback statutes. Incentive payments will be paid to an ACO, which includes hospitals and physicians, and the payments must be allocated among these parties. The final ACO regulations indicate that Medicare will not dictate how incentives are paid within the ACO, but the ACO must indicate the plan for incentives distribution in the application process. Thus, there should be substantial flexibility within the ACO to distribute incentives across participants, as long as they are set in advance.

This scenario also applies to allocation of losses; there needs to be an equitable plan outlined by the ACO. The final regulations added a requirement that the ACOs in Track 2 also establish reserves equal to 1% of per capita FFS Medicare Parts A & B expenditures for assigned beneficiaries. This amount should be determined based upon either expenditures from the most current performance year or the benchmark year.

In terms of the Stark Law and anti-kickback statutes, there is clearly a potential for the incentives payment in an ACO to implicate certain provisions within these regulations. CMS and the Office of Inspector General issued an "interim" final ruling on October 19, 2011, with a 60-day comment period regarding their position on anti-kickback statutes relative to ACOs. This subject is further discussed in under Legal Considerations in Chapter 7. Certain waivers have been established for CMS ACOs. This means that private ACOs are not covered under these waivers and will have to diligently establish their entities under the requirements of all antitrust and anti-kickback laws.

Physician productivity

The trend in the overall healthcare industry is an increase in physician employment by hospitals, and the concept of ACOs is playing no small role in this trend. Many hospitals feel the most effective way to accomplish the objective of an ACO is to develop a fully integrated healthcare delivery system, including a complete host of employed physicians.

When physicians are employed by hospitals, an incentive-based compensation model is typically in place. Currently, the trend is to pay physicians based on work-only value units, as established in the resource-based relative value scale, used by Medicare and many other payers to reimburse physicians for their professional services. Consequently, in most physician compensation arrangements, the key focus is on productivity, similar to the reimbursement model that currently exists. With reimbursement potentially changing to become more value-based, this inevitably must impact physician compensation arrangements so that incentives will be aligned. Still, physicians must maintain a baseline level of productivity at all times to ensure the employment arrangement is viable.

Similar to what is predicted for changes in reimbursement, the entire productivity-based compensation arrangement will not go away, but the portion of overall level of pay that is tied to productivity may begin to be reduced, with more being focused on overall management of service lines and outcome achievements. This is already occurring in some instances today, most notably in the specialties of orthopedics and cardiology, which have seen a substantial uptick in hospital employment. In many of these arrangements, a substantial portion of physicians' pay is being tied to management of the respective service lines. Within these management arrangements, compensation is tied to certain program milestones, various quality measures, patient and peer satisfaction, and cost control. As a result, the compensation model largely mirrors the concepts for ACOs.

These changes will likely persist as value-based payments continue to increase. Each specialty will see their compensation models change based on how reimbursement is modified for their specialty. Thus, while overall pay received may not necessarily decrease, it will likely be tied to more than just professional productivity.

Summary

The focus of this chapter has been to review historical and current reimbursement structures followed by an introduction to the reimbursement concepts that are on the horizon. The key point in this chapter is the potential shift of focus from one that is currently largely on volume (i.e., FFS) to one centered on quality (i.e., fee-for-value). There are definitely some positive results that come from this shift, but it is a substantial paradigm shift for the healthcare industry. Further, there are many challenges associated with such a change. Going forward, many details must be addressed to develop sustainable reimbursement models based on these premises for the future.

REFERENCES

1. Casto, Anne B. and Layman, PhD, Elizabeth. Principles of Healthcare Reimbursement. *http://library. ahima.org/xpedio/groups/public/documents/ahima/bok1_030575.pdf*. Accessed January 28, 2011.

2. Coker Group, Reimbursement Management: Improving the Success and Profitability of Your Practice. Chicago: American Medical Association, 2011. Page 3.

3. Morrison, Ian. Chasing Unicorns: The Future of ACOs. H&HN Weekly. *www.hhnmag.com/hhnmag_ app/jsp/articledisplay.jsp?dcrpath=HHNMAG%2FArticle%2Fdata%2F01JAN2011%2F010411HHN_ Weekly_Morrison&domain=HHNMAG*. Accessed January 11, 2011.

4. Overview of Bundled Payment. *www.randcompare.org/policy-options/bundled-payment*. Accessed January 28, 2011.

5. Paying for the Medical Home: Payment Models to Support Patient-Centered Medical Home Transformation in the Safety Net. *www.qhmedicalhome.org/safety-net/upload/SNMHI_ PolicyBrief_Issue1.pdf*. Accessed January 28, 2011.

6. Liethen, John. A Path to Accountable Care Runs Through the FTC. *www.dorsey.com/eupdate_liethen_health_ftc_april10/*. Accessed January 28, 2011.

7. Meershaert, John and Kieffer, Keith. Risk Models: Reimbursement Structure and Provider Payor Consultation. Foley's Physician-Hospital Alignment Series: A Critical Assessment of ACOs, Foley & Lardner LLP. Presented January 27, 2011.

Are You Ready for an ACO Environment?

You have read about the ACO requirements and anticipated changes. Now, for the difficult decision—do you want to join an ACO? Hospital administrators, physicians, practice managers, and other healthcare professionals can face this question. One of the first steps is to conduct a self-analysis to determine if you and/or your organization support the ACO philosophies. Would this be a good fit for you? What is the level of your current information technology (IT) infrastructure, technology adoption levels, and data collection capability? What is your current alignment of integration with a hospital; and if you are a hospital, with physicians?

Organizational Assessment

An organizational assessment can be determined by evaluating six key areas:

1.   The organizational and accountability level and culture

2.   Clinical results

3.   Infrastructure

4. Leadership: ability to embrace the ACO philosophy and lead a team into a patient-centered environment

5. Coordination and information-sharing abilities

6. Costs: what are actual costs at the diagnosis-related group (DRG) and current procedural terminology (CPT) level?

These categories must be assessed, and some level of competency is required before an organization should begin forming an ACO on its own. While an organization is assessing its capabilities, it should pay particular attention to:

• The operating data of the hospital

• The information regarding healthcare services in its area

• The availability for information sharing and coordination of care

• The relative acceptance level on the part of physicians and providers to participate in an ACO

• Current cost containment program

Physicians and physician groups need to assess the following:

• Current physician/hospital alignment

• IT infrastructure

• Cost at a CPT level

- Culture and philosophy

- Market (Medicare population, primary care physicians [PCP], and specialists in the area)

While conducting an assessment, an organization may choose to use surveys, focus groups, workshops, and one-on-one interviews as well as third-party objective groups who can come in to an organization and provide experience and a second opinion of the capabilities of an organization. As part of this assessment, organizations may find areas they can make improvements on right away, with or without the formation of an ACO.

As an organization begins to prepare for the ACO model to be launched by the Centers for Medicare & Medicaid Services (CMS), many executives are struggling with how to provide their administrative team, board members, and medical staff with accurate and relevant information that will help guide strategic decision-making, as well as information to evaluate the gaps as they relate to ACO development and implementation.

What is most notable here is that there is a shared recognition between hospitals and groups that they need to partner together to form ACOs and deliver account-able care. At the same time, however, a sorting out is underway that is very much geography-specific, differing from locality to locality.

The first key to a successful ACO is a strong alignment model with a hospital and other providers. If you currently have a well-established alignment with matching objectives and coordinated cultures, you may be a good candidate to participate in an ACO entity. Teamwork is essential in an ACO, and collaboration is mentioned throughout the ACO regulations. If you are not currently aligned, then perhaps you need to review that as a strategy.

Technology is another critical factor. The exchange of patient information between ACO participants is essential to meet the requirements of an ACO. Additionally, CMS has indicated that electronic connections with patients and their caregivers will be important as part of the delivery of care and customer service to the beneficiaries. Are you currently using an electronic health records (EHR) system that has been approved under Meaningful Use? If not, do you plan to implement one in 2012? Automation of data for patient records is significant and the ability to share the data within the ACO is a requirement.

Who are the appropriate players and leaders?

When forming an ACO, start by assessing the appropriate players:

- Your leadership

  - What is his or her vision?

  - Does he or she have the ability to successfully grasp all aspects of the ACO requirements and lead the group in this endeavor?

  - Does your leadership have the ability to create a team environment of full collaboration?

- Does the participating hospital have the ability to:

    - Deliver high-quality patient care?

    - Contain costs?

    - Be patient centered?

    - Collaborate with physicians and other healthcare providers?

- For physicians

    - Do they have the ability to work with competitors and become team members?

    - Do they have a reputation for delivering high-quality patient care?

    - Do they have the ability to control costs?

    - Can they be patient focused?

- Other providers

    - Do they have the ability to control costs?

    - Do they have a reputation for high-quality patient care?

    - Can they work together to be patient centered?

Financing—Startup and Ongoing Expenses

ACOs will require up-front costs. Among the most obvious is IT that will report and store data. Because all providers in an ACO will be jointly accountable for quality and cost measures, IT will have to be compatible for multiple providers to allow them to share information. Due to the high costs of IT, potential participants, such as small physician groups and solo practitioners, should assess whether joining an ACO is realistic. An ACO must have an IT infrastructure that enables it to collect, analyze, and share data among providers/suppliers in the ACO organization to support clinical decisions, as well as support CMS reporting. And the up-front costs may be greater than expected. Most early clinically integrated networks, which are precursors to ACOs, took longer than was anticipated to put in place and had greater than expected startup cost and staff requirements. Original ACO pilots were somewhat amazed at the high costs and extensive time required to build their IT infrastructure. Recently organized physician groups may also lack the history needed for benchmarking costs that would be required for a private ACO.

In addition to up-front costs, ACOs will require continuing expenses relating to reporting. These expenses will involve personnel, IT maintenance, governance, and continual coordination among the different members in an ACO. In an effort to assist providers with the upfront costs of creating a CMS ACO, the government has created a program called the Advance Payment Model. This model allows for three different payment options:

1. Upfront single fixed payment

2. Upfront, variable payment based on number of historically assigned beneficiaries

The Healthcare Executive's Guide to ACO Strategy

3. Monthly varying amount depending on number of historically assigned beneficiaries

These advance payments will be recovered from future savings distributed to the ACO—this is a loan, not a grant. Only two types of organizations will be eligible for the Advance Payment program. An ACO cannot include any inpatient facility and also must have less than $50 million in total annual revenue. The second type of ACO entity that could apply for financial assistance is one that does include inpatient facilities that are critical access hospitals and/or Medicare low-volume rural hospitals and has less than $80 million in total annual revenue. This program specifically excludes ACOs that are co-owned by a health plan, even if they fall into either of the above-mentioned categories. Also, only those ACOs that begin the ACO program in 2012 will be eligible to participate in the Advance Payment Model.

Organizations must make every effort to perform a detailed financial plan to establish capital requirements, milestones, and timing to include the following:

- Financial performance

  - Cash flow analysis and coverage

  - Cost analysis

- Future cash flow sustainability

- Projections: level of growth, improvements, staffing, costs, cash flow, etc.

- Market characteristics/fundamentals

- Capital requirements (Significant capital will be required to successful transform any organization into a medical home or ACO. Organizations must have a detailed financial plan to secure sufficient capital at the most favorable terms.)

- Project panel size insurance coverage (The organization must ensure that is has appropriate levels of malpractice insurance because it will be treating chronically ill Medicare patients.)

Market Assessment

The current market for ACOs is undergirded by lots of energy and buildup, and some pilot efforts are currently underway. CMS will limit the number of ACOs approved in a geographic location. The rapid growth of physician-hospital alignment over the last decade as reimbursements shrunk have forced physicians to look at other alternatives to protect their income. Also, managed care has created a payment system that rewards high technology procedures and providers who either own their own facilities or have increased their volume of services. Physicians are hiring consultants to help them create their own business models and are investing heavily in ancillary services and technology that will provide them with an annuitized income for years to come. The result is an increase in the direct competition between physicians and hospitals. For this reason, physicians are apt to resist ACOs.

Another market change is that physicians are starting to see that employment within a hospital is a viable model; therefore, the environment is increasingly collegial and collaborative. For years, physicians have competed against each other and would resist any acceptance of responsibility for care of all patients in a local delivery system such as an ACO where they do not control all of the factors.

Summary

In conclusion, ACOs offer physicians and hospitals a model to collaborate, innovate, and improve the quality of healthcare delivery in America, and share in the financial savings from those efforts. The ACO is intended to be a physician-based model as the PCP is the basis for assignment of beneficiaries to a CMS entity, and the PCP, as in most managed care programs, is responsible for directing and coordinating patient care. However, just like physician hospital organizations of the past, the model is only as good as the leaders and those in control of governance and decision-making. It is critical that physicians and hospitals take their time, investigate, and conduct proper due diligence before joining an ACO. Now is the time for physicians and hospitals to examine who they would like to integrate and collaborate with, and to approach and discuss these issues with colleagues. There will be many ACO options, and physicians need to understand how each option will affect their day-to-day practice of medicine, as well as the legal and financial implications. Each provider must also understand that the real focus of an ACO is "accountable care" and that means to the patient and the community. The patient must always come first for quality and customer service in any type of ACO model.

ACOs hold great promise as the healthcare delivery and payment system of the future. If the various demonstration projects prove the model to be successful, ACOs could be a groundbreaking change in the healthcare industry. Understandably, some healthcare providers are eager to be at the forefront of this movement and proceed quickly to participate in an ACO. However, despite the overwhelming amount of industry discussion and publication on this topic, there is still much concern by healthcare providers regarding the cost of participation and the ability to succeed in a CMS ACO environment. Therefore, we urge providers to take caution and carefully review the current statute and future regulatory guidelines before leaping into any new arrangements or making any changes to existing relationships.

CHAPTER

R

7

C H A P T E R

7

Legal Considerations

Disclaimer: The information in this chapter is not intended to be legal advice. This chapter is an overview of the legal structure and other considerations for a CMS ACO entity. It does not contain all legal requirements from the CMS ACO final regulations. For legal advice, readers should consult an attorney.

As part of the Patient Protection and Affordable Care Act (PPACA), the Secretary of Health and Human Services (the "Secretary") must establish a Shared Savings Program (SSP) that promotes accountability for patient care by groups of providers and coordinates services through an accountable care organization (ACO) no later than January 1, 2012.[1] In order to participate in the program, groups of providers and suppliers must work together to manage and create an eligible ACO that meets the requirements and quality standards of the Act and the Secretary to be eligible for payments and shared savings.

According to the Centers for Medicare & Medicaid Services (CMS), one of the most important healthcare delivery reforms contained in the Act is the encouragement of ACOs. CMS views ACOs as a way to "facilitate coordination and cooperation among providers to improve the quality of care for Medicare beneficiaries and reduce unnecessary costs."[2] Under the new §425.20 (Definitions), CMS defines an ACO as "a legal entity that is recognized and authorized under applicable State, Federal, or Tribal law, as identified by a Taxpayer Identification Number (TIN), and is formed by one or more ACO participant(s) that is(are) defined as §425.102(a) and may also include any other ACO participants described at §425.102(b).[3] The final regulations define an ACO participant as an individual or group of ACO provider(s)/supplier(s) that is identified by a Medicare-enrolled TIN, which alone or together with one or more other ACO participants comprise(s) an ACO, and that is included on the list of ACO participants that is required under §425.104(c)(5).[4]

In order to be eligible as an ACO, certain statutory requirements must be met. The Statute sets forth the minimum requirements to become an eligible ACO.[5] Under §425.102 of the final regulations, eligible providers and suppliers are defined as follows:

- ACO participants or combinations of ACO participants are eligible to form an ACO that may apply to participate in the Shared Savings Program include:

    - ACO professionals in group practice arrangements

    - Networks of individual practices of ACO professionals

    - Partnerships or joint venture arrangements between hospitals and ACO professionals

    - Hospitals employing ACO professionals

- Critical access hospitals (CAH) that bill under Method II (as described in §413.70(b)(3))

- Rural health clinics (RHC)

- Federally qualified health centers (FQHC)

- Other ACO participants that are not identified in the above list are eligible to participate through an ACO formed by one or more of the ACO participants identified in the above list

The CMS regulations define an ACO professional as an ACO provider/supplier who is either of the following:

- A physician legally authorized to practice medicine and surgery by the State in which he or she performs such activities

- A practitioner who is one of the following:

  - Physician assistant

  - Nurse practitioner

  - Clinical nurse specialist

An ACO provider/supplier must be enrolled in Medicare, bill for services and items to Medicare for fee-for-service (FFS) beneficiaries under a Medicare billing number assigned to a TIN of an ACO participant under the Medicare regulations, and be included on the list of ACO providers/suppliers submitted to CMS under the ACO entity.

Requirements

The list of requirements put forth by CMS is extensive and the regulations should be reviewed in their entirety by legal counsel for any healthcare provider considering formation of or joining an ACO. This section provides an overview of some of the key requirements for a CMS ACO:

- The ACO must have a minimum of 5,000 Medicare beneficiaries assigned to its entity

- It must be accountable for quality, cost, and overall care of Medicare FFS beneficiaries

- The entity must be a formal, legal structure under the laws of the state in which it is formed

- The ACO must sign a three-year agreement to participate (in some instances, the agreement will be beyond three years)

- The ACO must be able to receive/distribute shared savings and repay shared losses (losses under Track 2 only)

- The ACO must have a sufficient number of primary care physicians (PCP) to properly care for the assigned beneficiaries

- The ACO must be able to demonstrate that it meets patient-centeredness criteria

- The ACO must define its process for evidence-based medicine

- The ACO must have an infrastructure in place to collect, analyze, and report on quality and cost data[6]

Regardless of the form of collaboration used by the ACO, the parties must have established a mechanism for shared governance of the ACO. (Governance issues are discussed further in the next section.) The ACO also must have a leadership and management structure that includes clinical and administrative systems. This required clinical and financial integration also will be important with respect to antitrust considerations, which will be discussed later in this chapter.

The legal entity may be structured as a corporation, partnership, joint venture, limited liability company, foundation, or other entity permitted by state law. The requirement that the ACO be constituted as a legal entity and recognized under state, federal, or tribal law does not require existing legal entities to be appropriately recognized under state, federal, or tribal law to form a separate new entity for the purpose of participating in the program. Pursuant to the preamble, an existing legal entity that meets the ACO eligibility requirements under the regulations may operate as an ACO as long as it is recognized under applicable laws and satisfies all of the statutory and regulatory requirements related to ACOs.[7]

Striking the right balance between flexibility to encourage the development of the new innovative structures that may facilitate the success of ACOs and the need for some degree of certainty that the ACOs will withstand regulatory scrutiny is a challenge CMS faced in drafting the regulations. Significant investments will probably be necessary to form and implement ACOs; if the legal risks are perceived to be too high, ACOs will probably not be pursued as intended. Other federal agencies and departments, such as the Federal Trade Commission (FTC), the Office of Inspector General (OIG) of the Department of Health and Human Services (HHS), the Internal Revenue Service (IRS), and the Department of Justice (DOJ), have also played a significant role in the development of the CMS ACOs.

Governance

An ACO must have a mechanism for shared governance under the CMS program. Although this requirement may appear straightforward, depending on the types and number of ACO participants, it may prove to be one of the most challenging to accomplish. In a system of shared governance, not only are the participants accountable for a patient population, they also are accountable to each other. Through the governance structure, decisions will be made about payments to participating providers and suppliers, as well as all other financial and clinical aspects of the operation of the ACO. The greater the number and variety of ACO participants, the more challenging it will be to establish a governance structure that will be satisfactory to all of the participants. For example, an ACO may have the following as participants: multiple private practice groups of PCPs (enough to satisfy the statutory requirement discussed previously), multiple practice groups of various medical specialties, two or more hospitals (each of which with a large number of employed physicians), a network of private practice groups, and possibly other providers of services and suppliers. From a governance standpoint, how should these participants with diverse interests be organized to promote the best interest of the ACO?

Although much of the language from the proposed regulations was left in place for finalization of the law, some of the governance requirements were liberalized. In general, a CMS ACO must establish a governing body that has the authority to execute the functions of an ACO and must have responsibility for the oversight and strategic direction of the entity. The governing body members will be required to act consistent with the fiduciary responsibilities and duties. The governing body must also have a transparent governing process. As originally defined in the proposed law and then finalized in the regulations, each ACO must establish a governing body that is held by at least 75% of its ACO participants. However, under the final regulations, if an ACO chooses not to follow this rule, they must describe why they seek to be different and how the ACO will involve ACO participants in innovative ways for the ACO's governance. The regulations also require that at least one member of the governing body be a Medicare beneficiary who has no conflict of interest with the ACO or who has no immediate family member with a conflict of interest with the ACO (meaning that the beneficiary or an immediate family member cannot be a healthcare provider). The final ruling liberalized this section to say that if a Medicare beneficiary is *not* included on the governing body, the ACO must illustrate to CMS how it plans to provide for meaningful participation by Medicare beneficiaries in their governance.

The proposed regulations outlined stringent guidelines for establishment of the ACO governance; however, the final regulations give each ACO entity the latitude to structure their governing body. In their application, the ACO must clearly outline their governing body structure.

Implementation of some of these requirements may prove challenging. An important consideration, among many others, will be the concept of representation under the proposed rule and its impact on the fiduciary duties of members of the governing body under state corporate law. Under general corporate law, a member of the governing body of an ACO owes his or her duty to the ACO, not to any particular group or organization he or she represents under the proposed rule. Any ambiguity regarding fiduciary duties will likely increase the potential for conflicts of interest.

Also, consideration must be given to determining the means by which appropriate proportionate control by ACO participants will be achieved. Assuming a large number of ACO participants, the size of the board will be an important consideration. It may not be feasible for each participant to have direct representation on the board; some method of indirect representation may be necessary. Whether a participant is a for-profit provider or a nonprofit provider will also need to be considered for purposes of board representation. Sufficient representation of nonprofit providers must be assured consistent with their tax-exempt status. Keep in mind that CMS has not outlined strict rules in this area and, therefore, these decisions will be up to each ACO entity. Obtaining a consensus among the participants could be a challenge.

Comprehensive codes of conduct will be needed to promote ethical behavior, facilitate the execution of fiduciary duties, avoid conflicts of interest, and establish appropriate disclosure requirements. The potential for conflicting interests among ACO participants may be quite high, at least in the early stages of development. As the ACO moves toward a higher level of clinical and financial integration and, therefore, a greater alignment of interests, the potential for conflicts should be reduced.

The final rule contains significant additional requirements with respect to the leadership and management structure and the ACO's compliance plan. The ACO operations must be managed by an executive, officer, manager, general partner, or similar party whose appointment and removal are under the control of the ACO's governing body. A senior level medical director must provide oversight and clinical management to the entity. This physician must be one of the ACO participants who is physically present at a clinic or medical practice on a regular basis. The medical director must also be board-certified and licensed to practice in the state in which the ACO is operating.[8]

Antitrust Issues

A key element in the development of ACOs is integration, both financial and clinical. In order for ACOs to achieve the goals of providing better care to patients and lowering the costs of providing such care, a high degree of collaboration among providers is needed. The program requires integration, and the ACOs that do the best job of integrating as many aspects of their operation as possible will have the best chance of economic success. Although this is the goal of the statute, there are potential legal barriers, including other federal laws that could inhibit the development of ACOs. Among these are the antitrust laws. As discussed previously, many providers may come together to form an ACO, several of which may have been competitors. Such collaboration and consolidation among competitors that involves the anticompetitive fixing of prices or that leads to excessive market power may be illegal under the antitrust laws. That is, the components critical to the success of ACOs could make them impermissible under federal law and some state laws. Many providers have expressed concern about this apparent conflict and the uncertainty that the antitrust laws create when forming ACOs.

In addition to the anticompetitive price fixing concerns, there also are concerns about excessive market power, which could cause an ACO to run afoul of the antitrust laws. In other words, the larger in size that an ACO becomes and the greater percentage of the market that it occupies, the more anticompetitive it may become. By its sheer size and market power, an ACO's practices may become monopolistic, which may result in higher prices. This outcome also could subject the ACO to antitrust scrutiny.

The FTC and the Antitrust Division of the Department of Justice released a joint Final Policy Statement on October 21, 2011, regarding the antitrust enforcement policy related to ACOs participating in Medicare's SSP.[9] The originally proposed regulations contained a requirement for a mandatory antitrust review; the final policy removed this mandatory review requirement. However, the FTC and DOF policy statement said that, "The Agencies will vigilantly monitor complaints about an ACO's formation or conduct and take whatever enforcement action may be appropriate." The publication also emphasized that the CMS will work closely

with the FTC and DOF during the application process to review the formation
and participants of all CMS ACOs. CMS will also provide the Agencies with
aggregate claims data regarding allowed charges and FFS payments for all ACOs.
It should be noted that the final ACO regulations issued by HHS contain a
statement that approval by CMS of an ACO entity does not imply that the ACO
is in compliance with antitrust regulations. Each ACO is still responsible for
ensuring they do not violate any antitrust statutes. The Agencies' Final Policy
Statement only covers independent healthcare providers and provider groups who
join together to form an ACO. The Statement does not cover mergers or single,
fully integrated entities.

As with their previous publications regarding antitrust laws, these Agencies will
analyze an ACO to determine if there are price-fixing and market-allocation
agreements. Two of the key requirements for entities to avoid antitrust violations
are clinical integration and financial risk-sharing arrangements. Their policies
have been previously outlined in the Agencies' *Statements of Antitrust Enforcement Policy in Health Care* (a.k.a. "Health Care Statements"). One of the illus-
trations contained in the referenced Health Care Statements is related to joint
ventures. The Agencies state that clinical integration can be evidenced by the
venture implementing an "active and ongoing program to evaluate and modify
practice patterns by the venture's providers and to create a high degree of interdependence and cooperation among the providers to control costs and ensure
quality." This definition appears to fit directly within the ACO requirements.
Because the CMS ACO regulations allow for flexibility in establishment of
clinical management and entity governance, the Agencies will consider other
proposals for clinical integration as well.

The FTC and DOJ Policy Statement discusses two sections that further defines the Agencies' analysis of antitrust compliance. Section A outlines an antitrust safety zone and Section B identifies conduct that should be avoided by those ACOs that fall outside of the safety zone. This safety zone applies to ACOs participating in the CMS SSP only. It does not apply to private ACOs or other programs.

Below is an overview of the highlights of these sections. It is imperative that providers seek the services of an attorney for legal advice.

Section A: Antitrust safety zone for CMS ACO[10]

The ACOs that fall within the requirements of the antitrust safety zone will not be challenged by the Agencies, unless there are some extraordinary circumstances. For an ACO to fall within the safety zone, the independent ACO participants that provide the same service (referred to as a "common service") must have a combined share of 30% or less of each common service in each participant's primary service area (PSA). The PSA is defined as the lowest number of postal zip codes from which the ACO participant draws at least 75% of its patients. This must be calculated separately for each physician, each physician group practice, each inpatient facility, and each outpatient facility. Also, each hospital and ambulatory surgery center (ASC) must be non-exclusive to an ACO. Physicians can be exclusive (primary care) or non-exclusive to an ACO.

There is a rural exception if a provider exceeds the 30% PSA share. If the physician or physician group practice is a non-exclusive participant with an ACO and their primary office zip code is classified as "isolated rural" or "other small rural," they can qualify as a rural exception under the safety zone. A non-exclusive participating rural hospital may also qualify under this exception even if their PSA exceeds the 30% requirement. (The definition of the rural areas is further defined in the FTC/DOJ Final Policy Statement.)

Section B: ACOs outside of the safety zone [11]

ACOs that fall outside of the antitrust safety zone could still be considered lawful and precompetitive. ACOs that do not qualify under the safety zone need to avoid the following types of conduct:

- Improper sharing of competitively sensitive information

- Allowing private payers to incentivize or direct patients to choose certain providers

- Tying sales of ACO services to the private payer's purchase of other services from providers outside of the ACO, and vice versa

- Contracting on an exclusive basis with ACO physicians, hospitals, ASCs, or other providers, thereby preventing or discouraging them to contract with other entities outside of an ACO

- Restricting a private payer's ability to make available to its health plan enrollees cost, quality, or performance information to aid the enrollees in evaluating and selecting providers in the health plan, if that information is similar to the same measures used in the Shared Savings Program

The FTC and DOJ believe that providers seeking to create ACOs could benefit from additional guidance in the antitrust provisions. As a result, for CMS

ACO applicants, they have agreed to offer an expedited 90-day review for anti-trust guidance.

Stark Law and Anti-Kickback Statute

The federal physician self-referral law, also known as the Stark Law, prohibits a physician from referring patients for certain designated health services that are payable under Medicare or Medicaid to an entity with which the physician or an immediate family member of the physician has a financial relationship, including an ownership or compensation relationship, unless an exception under the law applies to the relationship.[12] Any entity that provides such referred services is prohibited from filing a claim with Medicare or billing any individual, third-party payer, or other entity for the services. The Stark Law, therefore, appears to be another potential legal obstacle to the formation and operation of ACOs. The high degree of integration that will be required for ACOs may result in many different types of financial relationships among physicians and hospitals that take into account quality improvement, efficiency, and cost savings considerations. These relationships may conflict with the Stark Law and other laws (such as the anti-kickback statute) intended to combat fraud and abuse.[13]

In conjunction with the release of the final ACO regulations, the OIG and CMS released an "interim final rule" on October 19, 2011, regarding possible waivers for CMS ACOs under portions of the Stark Law, anti-kickback statute, and certain civil monetary penalties. This ruling was released with a 60-day comment payment and as of the time this book was drafted, the final ruling had not been received due to the comment period.

Summary

This chapter has focused on some of the more significant legal considerations and regulations in the development of ACOs. The issues addressed here are by no means all of the legal issues that will need to be considered. Other legal issues to be considered include, but are not limited to, those arising from or related to: (1) Internal Revenue Service tax exempt laws and regulations, (2) health information privacy and security laws and regulations, and (3) state laws, such as those related to corporate practice of medicine, fee splitting, antitrust, fraud and abuse, insurance, and malpractice liability. In all matters involving legal considerations and issues, including those discussed in this chapter, it is critically important to consult a qualified attorney for specific legal advice.

REFERENCES

1. H.R. 3590 – Patient Protection and Affordable Care Act, Section 3022, 89.

2. *www.cms.gov.sharedsavingsprogram* (Overview) accessed 11/16/2011.

3. US Department of Health and Human Services, Centers for Medicare & Medicaid Services. Medicare Program; Medicare Shared Savings Program; Accountable Care Organizations. *Fed Reg.* 2011–27461; 42 *CFR* Part 425; [CMS-1345-F] RIN 0938-AQ22, 627.

4. Ibid.

5. Ibid., 632–633.

6. US Department of Health and Human Services, Centers for Medicare & Medicaid Services. Medicare Program; Medicare Shared Savings Program; Accountable Care Organizations. *Fed Reg.* 2011–27461; 42 *CFR* Part 425; [CMS-1345-F] RIN 0938-AQ22.

7. Ibid., 48, 52.

8. Ibid., 77.

9. Federal Trade Commission/Department of Justice, *Statement of Antitrust Enforcement, Policy Regarding Accountable Care Organizations Participating in the Medicare Shared Savings Program.*

10. Ibid., 6–9.

11. Ibid., 9–11.

12. Section 1877 of Social Security Act, enacted in 1989; 42 U.S.C. 1395.

13. Anti-Kickback Statute, 42 U.S.C.

The CMS Shared Savings Program

The Department of Health and Human Services (HHS), on behalf of the Centers for Medicare & Medicaid Services (CMS), released on October 20, 2011, the final regulations for the Shared Savings Program (SSP) under the CMS accountable care organization (ACO) model. Many of the proposed guidelines remained intact; however, numerous items were changed and in most cases, from the providers' perspective, the changes were an improvement. The design of the SSP places the patient in the center to focus on quality of care and delivery of excellent customer service. Providers are encouraged to include their patients in the decision-making of their healthcare.[1]

Although there are numerous sections to the final rule, this book focuses on four major areas: legal entity, benchmarks, quality measures, and the SSP provisions. In Chapter 7, we discussed the legal considerations and requirements for a CMS ACO entity. We discuss the benchmarks and beneficiary assignments within Chapter 9, and the quality measures are outlined in Chapter 10. This chapter provides an overview of the SSP and outlines how the savings (or losses) will be calculated. Our intent is to present an overview of the CMS program. Any provider who is interested in the CMS SSP should review the regulations or enlist legal counsel and/or a qualified healthcare consultant for assistance.

Program Overview

The SSP will now begin either on April 1 or July 1, 2012, rather than the previously announced January 1, 2012. For those ACOs with a start date of April 1, 2012, their first performance year will run for 21 months, through December 31, 2013. The second performance year will be January 1, 2014 through December 31, 2014; the third performance year will be for the period of January 1, 2015 through December 31, 2015. ACOs that begin the CMS program on July 1, 2012, will have their first performance year end on December 31, 2013, for a total of 18 months. Performance years two and three will be identical to those as the ACOs that start on April 1, 2012, which are calendar years 2014 and 2015.[2] As you can see, the 2012 ACOs will have a contract period that exceeds the originally proposed three years. It is anticipated that subsequent start dates will be for a three-year contract period.

When an ACO initially files for entry into the CMS program, it must submit the tax identification numbers (TIN) and national provider identifiers (NPI) of all participating providers/suppliers who are part of the ACO. Standard fee-for-service (FFS), diagnosis-related group (DRG), or per diem reimbursements will be paid directly to each provider as usual and will be unaffected by their ACO participation. Any shared savings will be paid directly to the TIN of the ACO.

The ACO entity is responsible for distributing the savings to each participating provider, and also for allocating any losses that must be repaid. CMS made no recommendation on how an ACO should distribute savings or allocate losses; however, they do require each ACO to submit a plan regarding their distribution methodology to be included with their application.[3]

Shared Savings Program Tracks

CMS has created two options for ACOs: a one-sided and a two-sided model. The one-sided model is referred to as Track 1. Under this model, ACOs are not financially responsible for any losses incurred for failure to reduce claim costs; they will share in any applicable savings. An ACO under Track 1 must move to Track 2 after their first contract period is complete. The maximum sharing rate under Track 1 is 50% based upon the maximum quality score. CMS has established a minimum savings rate (MSR) for both of their models. This minimum rate was created to ensure that the savings resulted from positive actions of the ACO participants and not just random results. It is anticipated that ACOs participating in Track 1 will be less experienced in the management of patient care in this type of setting. As a result, CMS created a MSR sliding scale under this track, ranging from 2% to 3.9% based upon the number of beneficiaries assigned to an ACO. This scale is shown in Figure 8.1.

FIGURE 8.1

MSR SLIDING SCALE FOR TRACK 1

NUMBER BENEFICIARIES	MSR (LOW END OF ASSIGNED BENEFICIARIES)	MSR (HIGH END OF ASSIGNED BENEFICIARIES)
5,000–5,999	3.9%	3.6%
6,000–6,999	3.6%	3.4%
7,000–7,999	3.4%	3.2%
8,000–8,999	3.2%	3.1%
9,000–9,999	3.1%	3.0%
10,000–14,999	3.0%	2.7%
15,000–19,999	2.7%	2.5%
20,000–49,999	2.5%	2.2%
50,000–59,999	2.2%	2.0%
60,000+	2.0%	

Source: US Department of Health and Human Services, Centers for Medicare & Medicaid Services. Medicare Program; Medicare Shared Savings Program: Accountable Care Organizations. Fed Reg. 2011-27461; 42 CFR Part 425; [CMS-1345-F] RIN 0938-AQ22, 464.

ACOs in Track 1 that successfully meet the quality measures and all other requirements will be eligible to receive shared savings on the first dollar of savings after the applicable MSR has been met.[4] Track 2, also called the two-sided model, requires ACOs to share in both savings and losses. For 2012, it is anticipated that those groups who have experience in patient-centered care and evidence-based medicine will enroll in the Track 2 model as it also allows for a greater shared savings opportunity. Under this model, the maximum sharing rate is 60% based

The Healthcare Executive's Guide to ACO Strategy

upon the maximum quality score. The minimum savings rate for Track 2 is a flat 2%.[5]

If the per capita cost per beneficiary is 2% or more above the cost benchmark, Track 2 ACOs must pay back a portion of their losses. A ceiling on losses has been set at 60%, which matches the maximum savings. However, CMS has established a cap for shared losses for each of the first performance years so that an ACO is not financially devastated with a large repayment. Those caps are outlined below:[6]

- 5.0%—1st year

- 7.5%—2nd year

- 10%—3rd year

If an ACO is required to pay back a loss, they must do so in full within 60 days from the date of notification. ACOs participating under Track 2 must at the time of application, and annually subsequent to that, indicate to CMS what repayment mechanism has been established for any possible losses.[7]

ACOs that successfully complete their first agreement period under Track 2 without a loss may apply for a second agreement period. ACOs that successfully complete their first agreement period under Track 1 without a loss will be moved to Track 2 for their second agreement period; they cannot remain under Track 1 beyond their first contract period. Figure 8.2 provides the key elements of the SSP models at a glance.

FIGURE 8.2

SHARED SAVINGS PROGRAM SUMMARY AND BENCHMARKS

PROGRAM ELEMENT	TRACK 1: ONE-SIDED MODEL	TRACK 2: TWO-SIDED MODEL
Maximum sharing rate	50%	60%
Minimum savings rate (MSR)	Varies by population; see Figure 8.1	Flat 2%
Maximum sharing cap	10% of ACO's Benchmark	15% of ACO's Benchmark
Shared savings	First dollar once MSR is met	First dollar once MSR is met
Minimum loss rate (MLR)	n/a	2%
Shared losses	n/a	One minus final sharing rate once minimum loss rate has been met; not to exceed 60%

Source: Coker Group.

ACOs with a net loss during their first agreement period may continue to participate if they meet all other requirements. However, such continued participation will only be allowed under the Track 2 option. In this situation, the ACO must identify what safeguards are in place to prevent further losses in the second period.[8]

Interim Payment Option

ACOs that begin in 2012 will have a first performance year that exceeds 12 months because the first year will be either 21 or 18 months in duration, depending upon the April 1 or July 1, 2012, startup date. To again assist participants with managing their expenses, CMS is offering an Interim Payment Option for ACOs that start in 2012 only. This option will allow them to receive a shared savings payment based upon their first 12 months of performance, with quality performance retroactive to January 1, 2012, if they qualify, with a final reconciliation occurring at the end of the ACO's first performance year.[9] Track 1 ACOs that opt for the interim payment must request such at the time of their application and must also demonstrate their repayment mechanism in the event of an overpayment under the SSP. (Track 2 ACOs are already required to document their repayment mechanism since they are accountable for losses under their model.)

As mentioned previously, ACOs requesting an interim payment will have their quality performance based upon group practice reporting option (GPRO) quality data reported for calendar year 2012. CMS believes that quality data based on 2012 is an appropriate measure of the ACO's performance because ACOs for that year will have submitted GPRO date for calendar year 2012 as part of demonstrating their eligibility for the 2012 Physician Quality Reporting System (PQRS) incentive. CMS will use the historical benchmark that will be updated for beneficiary risk for the first 12 months to determine the cost benchmark.[10] December 31, 2013, will end the first performance year for the 2012 ACO entities and reconciliation will be based upon that entire performance period. The final rule details the reconciliation methodology on pp. 518–519 in the October 20, 2011, document. (**Note:** the Interim Payment Option should not be confused with the Advance Payment Model. That model is limited to only two types of organizations and is an advance to assist with startup expenditures.)

Summary

CMS received thousands of comments in 2011 after release of the proposed ACO regulations. In response to the concerns from providers and professional organizations regarding the financial burden and lack of incentives to participate, HHS and CMS have made numerous attempts to make their ACO program more attractive to physicians, hospitals, and other healthcare providers. They expanded the assignment of beneficiaries to include nurse practitioners, physician assistants, and clinical nurse specialists; they eliminated the 25% withhold, increased the performance payment limit, and added federally qualified health centers and rural health clinics to the list of organizations that could form an ACO. They also included adjustments to the benchmarks for new beneficiaries and for beneficiaries with certain risk factors. One of the key elements that CMS has promised is faster feedback to ACOs regarding claim data (a three-month claims run-out rather than a six-month run-out) to enable them to better monitor their performance. They also reduced the quality measures to 33, down from 65 measures in the proposed regulations.

Some elements are still being finalized as of the end of 2011 regarding benchmarks and quality sharing rates. All items should be resolved in early 2012 because the first CMS ACO will go live April 1, 2012.

REFERENCES

1. US Department of Health and Human Services, Centers for Medicare & Medicaid Services. Medicare Program; Medicare Shared Savings Program: Accountable Care Organizations. *Fed Reg.* 2011-27461; 42 *CFR* Part 425; [CMS-1345-F] RIN 0938-AQ22, page 15.

2. Ibid., 130.

3. Ibid., 55.

4. Ibid., 125, 397.

5. Ibid., 397.

6. Ibid., 398.

7. Ibid., 509.

8. Ibid., 394.

9. Ibid., 515.

10. Ibid., 516–517.

Benchmarks for CMS Shared Savings Program

One of the main objectives of accountable care organizations (ACO) is to attain a higher quality of care at a lower cost. This means effective measures must be in place to begin to quantify, track, and compare data sets internally as well as to external resources. The ACO concept will only succeed if organizations pledge to not cut costs at the expense of quality, safety, and patient satisfaction. Simply, do services rendered meet the needs of patients and customers, and how do the patients feel about it? From the perspective of the Centers for Medicare & Medicaid Services (CMS), the cost must come in below a certain benchmark in order to be eligible for shared savings. Even if quality measures are met, failure to meet the cost goals could require the ACO to pay losses to CMS under Track 2. This is a real concern to many providers since they know that to establish an ACO entity under the CMS model will cost money. CMS will not take into account any "corporate" or ACO structural costs; they will only analyze the costs of medical care. However, the healthcare provider participants do care about startup costs and ongoing management cost and will be very concerned if they are required to share in loss repayments back to Medicare.

Assignment of Beneficiaries

The final regulations detail how the benchmarks for costs will be established. This benchmark is the cost per beneficiary (per capita) the ACO must fall below in order to earn any shared savings during a performance year. In order to determine a benchmark, CMS must first assign beneficiaries to an ACO. The methodology will use the beneficiary's primary care provider (PCP) to determine the assignment. If a PCP is participating in an ACO, all of his or her Medicare patients will be assigned to their respective ACO based on the guidelines outlined below. For purposes of the CMS ACO, primary care is defined as family medicine, general practice, internal medicine, or geriatric medicine.[1] Eligible PCPs include physicians, nurse practitioners, physician assistants, and clinical nurse specialists.

In order to properly assign a PCP to a beneficiary based on the plurality of care, CMS has identified a list of codes from the healthcare common procedure coding system (HCPCS) to be used to define primary care services. These codes are the following:

- 99201–99215

- 99304–99350

- G0402, G0438, and G0439[2]

CMS will develop a crosswalk for HCPCS codes to certain revenue codes for federally qualified health centers (FQHC) and rural health clinics (RHC) to ensure their services are included in the review of PCP services. They will use revenue codes 0521, 0522, 0524, and 0525.

In the event that a beneficiary is not seeing a PCP, assignment will be based on the plurality of care rendered by a specialist for primary care services. One example of this is a patient with a chronic cardiac disease. A cardiologist may manage routine primary care services for a given patient in addition to specific services for heart care.[3]

Beneficiaries will be assigned prospectively to an ACO based on 12 months of the most recent claim data that identifies their respective PCP. This data will be updated quarterly to add or delete beneficiaries based on claims data. CMS outlined a new "step-wise" approach for this process.[4] It includes the HCPCS codes, plurality of care, type of provider, and physician specialty. Final beneficiary assignment will be reconciled at the end of each performance year based on actual data from that year. CMS has made a commitment to immediately provide the ACOs with beneficiary identification upon their entry into the program. Under the final regulations, CMS liberalized their previous guidelines and will now allow ACOs to contact beneficiaries directly to advise them of their assignment to an ACO. The ACO can then advise the Medicarees of its intent to obtain the beneficiaries' claim data for the program. If the beneficiary does not decline data sharing within 30 days, the ACO can request the respective claim data from CMS.[5]

Cost Benchmarks

Once beneficiaries have been identified for specific ACOs, CMS will calculate the respective cost benchmark for each ACO. To establish the initial benchmark,

CMS will use the previous three years of data based on Parts A and B fee-for-service claims. Each of the three prior years (called a benchmark year or "BY") will be weighted as follows:[6]

- Benchmark Year 1 = 10%

- Benchmark Year 2 = 30%

- Benchmark Year 3 = 60%

Because year three is the most recent year of data, it will have the highest weight assigned to determine the total benchmark for the ACO reporting year. For ACOs that are established in 2012, that year will begin the first performance year and years 2009, 2010, and 2011 will be used as the data benchmark years. CMS will add the following risk factors cost categories when calculating historical expenditures:[7]

- End-stage renal disease (ESRD)

- Disabled

- Aged/dual eligibility for Medicare/Medicaid

- Aged/non-dual eligibility for Medicare/Medicaid

Expenditures will be adjusted for severity and case mix using the CMS Hierarchical Condition Category (HCC) scores. To evaluate performance and provide feedback to the ACOs, CMS has committed to timelier reporting and will use a three-month claims run-out period. This will give the ACO entities quarterly updates with the most recent data available. Additionally, CMS will update beneficiary data as new beneficiaries will be added as they become Medicare eligible or when existing Medicare beneficiaries incur primary care services and become assigned to an ACO. Claim data for these newly assigned beneficiaries will be adjusted using HCC. Data for beneficiaries already assigned to an ACO (referred to as "continuously assigned beneficiary") will be adjusted for each performance year using demographics, unless the HCC deems a lower risk score.[8]

CMS will conduct a final reconciliation retrospectively of assigned beneficiaries to an ACO based on claim data of actual use of the beneficiary's PCP alignment. Any beneficiaries that did not complete the entire performance year in the assigned ACO will be removed from the calculation of performance. This will not penalize the ACO if it did not manage the entire period of care for a given beneficiary if they moved out of the area or were no longer receiving a plurality of care from a participating PCP.[9]

At the beginning of the three-year ACO contract period, CMS will make the calculations described above for performance year one, and that will be the cost goal for the ACO. For example, if the adjusted per capita benchmark is $8,000, the ACO's goal is to keep medical costs to $8,000 or less for each beneficiary in their service area. If there is a loss, the losses are capped each year to minimize a financial burden to the participating providers within the ACO participating under Track 2. The first year has a cap of 5%, the second year is capped at 7.5%, and the third year has a maximum loss repayment of 10%.[10]

It is essential that an ACO participating in the CMS program manage all patients under the quality and cost requirements, as it cannot be sure which beneficiaries will end up in its assigned pool. For example, in year one, a 64-year old may receive treatment by one or more of the providers in an ACO and his or her claim experience would not be included in that first year. However, when he or she turns 65 years old in year two of the ACO contract, his or her Medicare claims data would then be assigned to an ACO based on his or her participating PCP. Also, Medicare recipients may choose to change their PCP during a given year, or they may move, and they will be assigned to a CMS ACO based on the greatest volume of services (plurality) rendered by a participating PCP. It is also important to note that ACOs may not avoid at-risk patients. If CMS determines that an ACO has taken steps to avoid such patients (thus likely reducing their exposure to increasing or high costs), CMS may impose sanctions on the ACO, including termination from the program.

Summary

The biggest challenge is that under the current process of reimbursement, the ACO makes no legitimate business sense in today's system that rewards productivity, ordering tests, and admitting patients to the hospital. Clearly, the future will require a focus on quality, outcomes, patient safety, patient satisfaction, and cost management—it is just a matter of time. The purpose of this book is to help the reader strive to achieve similar goals and objectives of the organizations referenced here.

REFERENCES

1. U.S. Department of Health and Human Services, Centers for Medicare & Medicaid Services. Medicare Program; Medicare Shared Savings Program: Accountable Care Organizations. *Fed Reg.* 2011-27461; 42 *CFR* Part 425; [CMS-1345-F] RIN 0938-AQ22, page number 27, 34, 201

2. Ibid., 218

3. Ibid.

4. Ibid., 202, 209–210, 244

5. Ibid., 185

6. Ibid., 417, 420

7. Ibid., 420

8. Ibid., 427–429

9. Ibid., 232–234

10. Ibid., 398

Quality Measures

In 2001, the Institute of Medicine released their widely publicized position paper, "Crossing the Quality Chasm: A New Health System for the 21st Century," which stated that there was a definitive chasm "between the healthcare we have and the healthcare we should have."[1] As a result of that publication and an overall shift within the healthcare industry, over the past decade an increased focus on patient-centered care, quality, and outcomes has occurred. This increased concentration on the quality aspect of medicine has been accomplished through many different pay-for-performance programs, the Physician Quality Reporting System (PQRS, formerly PQRI), and demonstration programs from private payers. Whereas these programs began to increase the focus on quality within the industry, accountable care organizations (ACO) will build on this focus by bringing quality to the forefront of the delivery of healthcare. This chapter discusses the quality measures defined in the final Centers for Medicare & Medicaid Services (CMS) regulations and evidence-based outcomes.

Benchmarks, Standardization, and Protocols

Comparing provider performance to clinical benchmarks, using standardized treatment plans, and developing medical protocols are not novel practices within the healthcare industry, but they will take a new role within the ACO structure. The goal of the CMS ACO program is to improve quality of care for individuals, improve overall health for the population, and reduce healthcare expenditures. Medicare has attempted to address the improved care with quality measures outlined in their final regulations. The good news for all providers interested in joining or starting a CMS ACO is that the quality measures were reduced from the proposed number of 65 down to 33 measures. Based on the comments received during the review period in 2011, CMS wanted to minimize the efforts required by providers to measure and report upon quality required under the program. However, it was also important to use measures that brought value to the care of beneficiaries. As a result, CMS has adopted quality measures that have been tested, validated, and clinically accepted. Most of the quality measures they have finalized have been endorsed by the National Quality Forum. The corresponding NQF number is shown in the measures for reference. However, CMS did not choose only NQF-endorsed measures.

The final quality measures are divided into four domains: Patient/Caregiver Experience, Care Coordination/Patient Safety, Preventive Health, and At-Risk Population. The At-Risk Population measures focus on diabetes, hypertension, ischemic vascular disease, heart failure, and coronary artery disease. CMS has assigned points to each of the categories, with double points assessed for electronic health records (EHR). Figure 10.1 illustrates the points by category.

FIGURE 10.1

TOTAL POINTS BY QUALITY DOMAIN

DOMAIN	TOTAL INDIVIDUAL MEASURES (TABLE F1)	TOTAL MEASURES FOR SCORING PURPOSES	TOTAL POTENTIAL POINTS PER DOMAIN	DOMAIN WEIGHT
Patient/ caregiver experience	7	One measure with six survey module measures combined, plus one individual measure	4	25%
Care coordination/ Patient safety	6	Six measures, plus the EHR measure double-weighted (4 points)	14	25%
Preventative health	8	Eight measures	16	25%
At-risk population	12	Seven measures, including five component diabetes composite measures and two component CAD composite measures	14	25%
Total	**33**	**23**	**48**	**100%**

Source: *U.S. Department of Health and Human Services, Centers for Medicare & Medicaid Services. Medicare Program; Medicare Shared Savings Program: Accountable Care Organizations. Fed Reg. 2011-27461; 42 CFR Part 425; [CMS-1345-F] RIN 0938-AQ22, 358.*

Figure 10.2 details the 33 quality measures outlined in the final CMS regulations. The chart includes how the data is to be submitted/collected (survey, claims, group practice reporting option [GPRO] interface, etc.) and also by year if it is a reported measure or performance-based measure. Seven of the measures will be collected via patient surveys, three will be calculated from actual claims, 22 will be obtained from the GPRO Web interface, and one will be received via the EHR Incentive Program data. All quality measures will have a 12-month calendar year reporting period regardless of the ACO start date. Also, an added bonus for the participating providers is that CMS will fund the administration of the patient experience surveys for 2012 and 2013. ACOs will then have to select a survey vendor from a CMS-approved list and pay for report administration and results for 2014 and beyond.

CMS is establishing national benchmarks for quality using national samplings of Medicare fee-for-service (FFS) claim data and Medicare Advantage (MA) quality data. They will use a flat percentage if FFS claims and MA quality data are unavailable. They chose to establish national benchmarks rather than regional ones because the FFS program is at a national level. Their goal is to measure quality improvement and make comparisons over time between FFS and ACO populations at a national level. ACOs must meet the quality goals annually in order to receive monies under the Shared Savings Program (SSP). The regulations require that each ACO must achieve the quality performance standard on 70% of the measures in *each* domain. If the EHR measure is not completely and accurately recorded, an ACO could miss the 70% minimum requirement for that segment because the EHR measure is valued at double points. If an ACO scores zero for an entire domain, it would not be eligible for any shared savings. Figure 10.3 identifies how points will be assessed using the FFS or MA rate.

FIGURE 10.2

CMS SHARED SAVINGS QUALITY MEASURES

| DOMAIN | MEASURE TITLE | NQF MEASURE #/ MEASURE STEWARD | METHOD OF DATA SUBMISSION | PAY FOR PERFORMANCE PHASE IN | | |
| | | | | R = REPORTING | P = PERFORMANCE | |
				PERFORMANCE YEAR 1	YEAR 2	YEAR 3
AIM: Better Care for Individuals						
1. Patient/Caregiver experience	CAHPS: Getting timely care, appointments, and information	NQF #5 AHRQ†	Survey	R	P	P
2. Patient/Caregiver experience	CAHPS: How well your doctors communicate	NQF #5 AHRQ	Survey	R	P	P
3. Patient/Caregiver experience	CAHPS: Patients' ranking of doctor	NQF #5 AHRQ	Survey	R	P	P
4. Patient/Caregiver experience	CAHPS: Access to specialists	NQF #5 AHRQ	Survey	R	P	P
5. Patient/Caregiver experience	CAHPS: Health promotion and education	NQF #5 AHRQ	Survey	R	P	P
6. Patient/Caregiver experience	CAHPS: Shared decision-making	NQF #5 AHRQ	Survey	R	P	P
7. Patient/Caregiver experience	CAHPS: Health status/ Functional status	NQF #6 AHRQ	Survey	R	R	R
8. Care coordination/ Patient safety	Risk-standardized, all-condition readmission*	NQF #TBD CMS	Claims	R	R	P

FIGURE 10.2

CMS SHARED SAVINGS QUALITY MEASURES (CONT.)

DOMAIN	MEASURE TITLE	NQF MEASURE #/ MEASURE STEWARD	METHOD OF DATA SUBMISSION	PAY FOR PERFORMANCE PHASE IN R = REPORTING P = PERFORMANCE		
				PERFORMANCE YEAR 1	YEAR 2	YEAR 3
AIM: Better Care for Individuals (cont.)						
9. Care coordination/ Patient safety	Ambulatory sensitive conditions admissions: Chronic obstructive pulmonary disease (AHRQ prevention quality indicator [PQI] #5)	NQF #275 AHRQ	Claims	R	P	P
10. Care coordination/ Patient safety	Ambulatory sensitive conditions admissions: Congestive heart failure (AHRQ prevention quality indicator [PQI] #8)	NQF #277 AHRQ	Claims	R	P	P
11. Care coordination/ Patient safety	Percent of PCPs who successfully qualify for an EHR incentive program payment	CMS	EHR Incentive program reporting	R	P	P
12. Care coordination/ Patient safety	Medication reconciliation: Reconciliation after discharge from an inpatient facility	NQF #97 AMA-PCPI†/ NCQA†	GPRO Web interface	R	P	P
13. Care coordination/ Patient safety	Falls: Screening for fall risk	NQF #101 NCQA	GPRO Web interface	R	P	P

The Healthcare Executive's Guide to ACO Strategy

FIGURE 10.2
CMS SHARED SAVINGS QUALITY MEASURES (CONT.)

| DOMAIN | MEASURE TITLE | NQF MEASURE #/ MEASURE STEWARD | METHOD OF DATA SUBMISSION | PAY FOR PERFORMANCE PHASE IN | | |
| | | | | R = REPORTING | P = PERFORMANCE | |
				PERFORMANCE YEAR 1	YEAR 2	YEAR 3
14. Preventive health	Influenza immunization	NQF #41 AMA-PCPI	GPRO Web interface	R	P	P
15. Preventive health	Pneumococcal vaccination	NQF #43 NCQA	GPRO Web interface	R	P	P
16. Preventive health	Adult weight screening and follow-up	NQF #421 CMS	GPRO Web interface	R	P	P
17. Preventive health	Tobacco use assessment and tobacco cessation intervention	NQF #28 AMA-PCPI	GPRO Web interface	R	P	P
18. Preventive health	Depression screening	NQF #418 CMS	GPRO Web interface	R	P	P
19. Preventive health	Colorectal cancer screening	NQF #34 NCQA	GPRO Web interface	R	R	P
20. Preventive health	Mammography screening	NQF #31 NCQA	GPRO Web interface	R	R	P
21. Preventive health	Proportion of adults 18+ who had their blood pressure measured with the preceding two years	CMS	GPRO Web interface	R	R	P

FIGURE 10.2
CMS SHARED SAVINGS QUALITY MEASURES (CONT.)

DOMAIN	MEASURE TITLE	NQF MEASURE #/ MEASURE STEWARD	METHOD OF DATA SUBMISSION	PAY FOR PERFORMANCE PHASE IN		
				R = REPORTING	P = PERFORMANCE	
				PERFORMANCE YEAR 1	YEAR 2	YEAR 3
AIM: Better Health for Populations (cont.)						
22. At-risk population—Diabetes	Diabetes composite (all or nothing scoring): Hemoglobin A1c control (<8%)	NQF #0729 MN Community measurement	GPRO Web interface	R	P	P
23. At-risk population—Diabetes	Diabetes composite (all or nothing scoring): Low-density lipoprotein (<100)	NQF #0729 MN Community measurement	GPRO Web interface	R	P	P
24. At-risk population—Diabetes	Diabetes composite (all or nothing scoring): Blood pressure <140/90	NQF #0729 MN Community measurement	GPRO Web interface	R	P	P
25. At-risk population—Diabetes	Diabetes composite (all or nothing scoring): Tobacco non-use	NQF #0729 MN Community measurement	GPRO Web interface	R	P	P
26. At-risk population—Diabetes	Diabetes composite (all or nothing scoring): Aspirin use	NQF #0729 MN Community measurement	GPRO Web interface	R	P	P

The Healthcare Executive's Guide to ACO Strategy

FIGURE 10.2
CMS SHARED SAVINGS QUALITY MEASURES (CONT.)

DOMAIN	MEASURE TITLE	NQF MEASURE #/ MEASURE STEWARD	METHOD OF DATA SUBMISSION	PAY FOR PERFORMANCE PHASE IN R = REPORTING P = PERFORMANCE		
				PERFORMANCE YEAR 1	YEAR 2	YEAR 3
27. At-risk population— Diabetes	Diabetes mellitus: Hemoglobin A1c poor control (>9%)	NQF #59 NCQA	GPRO Web interface	R	P	P
28. At-risk population— Hypertension	Hypertension (HTN): Blood pressure control	NQF #18 NCQA	GPRO Web interface	R	P	P
29. At-risk population— Ischemic vascular disease	Ischemic vascular disease (IVD): Complete lipid profile and LDL control <100 mg/dl	NQF #75 NCQA	GPRO Web interface	R	P	P
30. At-risk population— Ischemic vascular disease	Ischemic vascular disease (IVD): Use of aspirin or another antithrombotic	NQF #68 NCQA	GPRO Web interface	R	P	P
31. At-risk population— Heart failure	Heart failure: Beta-blocker therapy for left ventricular systolic dysfunction (LVSD)	NQF #83 AMA-PCPI	GPRO Web interface	R	R	P
32. At-risk population— Coronary artery disease	Coronary artery disease (CAD) composite: All or nothing scoring: Drug therapy for lowering LDL-cholesterol	NQF #74 CMS (composite)/ AMA-PCPI (individual component)	GPRO Web interface	R	R	P

FIGURE 10.2

CMS SHARED SAVINGS QUALITY MEASURES (CONT.)

DOMAIN	MEASURE TITLE	NQF MEASURE #/ MEASURE STEWARD	METHOD OF DATA SUBMISSION	PAY FOR PERFORMANCE PHASE IN		
				R = REPORTING	P = PERFORMANCE	
				PERFORMANCE YEAR 1	YEAR 2	YEAR 3

AIM: Better Health for Populations (cont.)

DOMAIN	MEASURE TITLE	NQF MEASURE #/ MEASURE STEWARD	METHOD OF DATA SUBMISSION	PERFORMANCE YEAR 1	YEAR 2	YEAR 3
33. At-risk population— Coronary artery disease	Coronary artery disease (CAD) composite: All or nothing scoring: Angiotensin-converting enzyme (ACE) inhibitor or angiotensin receptor blocker (ARB) therapy for patients with CAD and diabetes and/or left ventricular systolic dysfunction (LVSD)	NQF #66 CMS (composite)/ AMA-PCPI (individual component)	GPRO Web interface	R	R	P

*We note that this measure has been under development and that finalization of this measure is contingent upon the availability of measures specifications before the establishment of the Shared Savings Program on January 1, 2012.

†AMA-PCPI— American Medical Association convened Physician Consortium for Performance Improvement®

†AHRQ- Agency for Healthcare Research and Quality

†NCQA- National Committee for Quality Assurance

Source: U.S. Department of Health and Human Services, Centers for Medicare & Medicaid Services. Medicare Program; Medicare Shared Savings Program: Accountable Care Organizations. Fed Reg. 2011-27461; 42 CFR Part 425; [CMS-1345-F] RIN 0938-AQ22, 324-326

FIGURE 10.3

ACO PERFORMANCE-LEVEL QUALITY POINTS: SLIDING SCALE MEASURE SCORING

ACO PERFORMANCE LEVEL	QUALITY PTS	EHR PTS
90+ percentile FFS/MA Rate or 90+ percent	2	4
80+ percentile FFS/MA Rate or 80+ percent	1.85	3.7
70+ percentile FFS/MA Rate or 70+ percent	1.7	3.4
60+ percentile FFS/MA Rate or 60+ percent	1.55	3.1
50+ percentile FFS/MA Rate or 50+ percent	1.4	2.8
40+ percentile FFS/MA Rate or 40+ percent	1.25	2.5
30+ percentile FFS/MA Rate or 30+ percent	1.1	2.2
<30 percentile FFS/MA Rate or < 30 percent	No Points	

Source: *U.S. Department of Health and Human Services, Centers for Medicare & Medicaid Services. Medicare Program; Medicare Shared Savings Program: Accountable Care Organizations.* Fed Reg. 2011-27461; 42 CFR Part 425; [CMS-1345-F] RIN 0938-AQ22, 357–358 .

Use of Evidence-Based Medicine

Widespread use of evidence-based medicine will be required in order for ACOs (private or Medicare) to deliver quality care. The final CMS regulations state that ACOs participating in the CMS program must define processes that promote evidence-based medicine and patient engagement. Evidence-based outcomes are discussed throughout the regulations. Although practicing evidence-based medicine seems an obvious course of action, in current practice this is not often the case. There are significant barriers to the practice of evidence-based medicine, including:

- Time pressures

- Perceived threats to autonomy

- Preference for "colloquial" knowledge based on individual experiences

- Difficulty in accessing the evidence base

- Difficulty differentiating useful and accurate evidence from the inaccurate or inapplicable

- Lack of resources[2]

Thus, although many providers agree that evidence-based medicine is currently important, they do not necessarily follow this process because of these difficulties. However, under an ACO model, the barriers relative to evidence-based medicine either will need to be overcome with support that comes from the structure of the model itself or by the providers' own volition.

Impact of standardization and protocols

In addition to evidence-based medicine, use of standardized clinical practices or medical protocols may also be included as part of an ACO structure as a way to help drive quality. Protocols can be defined as "a set of predetermined criteria that define appropriate [medical staff] interventions that articulate or describe situations in which the [medical staff member] makes judgments relative to a course of action for effective management of common patient care problems."[3] The use of protocols historically has been debated within the healthcare industry largely because of concern that protocols do not provide adequate parameters to assist medical staff in acting on the requisite treatment.[4] However, use of protocols has been gaining favor within the medical community, largely because it creates a baseline for clinical care. Thus, in the absence of other confounding factors, a protocol would ensure a minimum standard of quality, safe care. This would likely be one impetus for the inclusion of protocol-driven medicine within the ACO model.

Although the creation of protocols could occur on a national level (i.e., protocols would be developed that would then apply to and be used by all ACOs), it is also possible that individual ACOs will be allowed to create their own set of protocols. In either case, it is likely that professional medical organizations (e.g., the American Academy of Family Physicians, the American College of Cardiology, the American Diabetes Association, etc.) may be leveraged to assist in the development of applicable protocols.

Measuring Outcomes

Even though the healthcare industry is still, to a large degree, focused on production (the "churn and burn" method of medicine is pervasive, and physicians are still incented to generate higher volumes, rather than improved outcomes), under ACOs the standard will not be production, but quality. Thus, rather than provider performance being benchmarked by patient visits or number of encounters, it will be benchmarked against outcome scores for specific illnesses and adherence to best clinical practices.

There are several important components relative to measuring outcomes under an ACO model:

1. Everyone and everything should be measured. Quality reporting programs currently in place have typically included a threshold for patient reporting (e.g., in PQRS, many measures require reporting on 80% of applicable patients seen within the practice). For a number of reasons (e.g., death, relocation outside of the service area, patient discharge from practice, etc.), not all patients will be measured throughout their treatment process. Therefore, all patients should be measured across all metrics to ensure the reporting threshold can be met.

2. The use of scorecards will likely be necessary to appropriately measure outcomes. In many healthcare organizations, key performance indicators are measured and tracked on a routine basis using scorecards. The scorecards are typically able to provide performance feedback by provider, by service line, or for the organization as a whole on individual or aggregated metrics. Under an ACO model, the same would need to be true so that outcomes can be assessed on both a micro and macro level, and performance feedback could be used to modify or strengthen specific practice patterns. This consistent, timely feedback will be important to providers so they are able to track their performance and make adjustments within a reporting cycle, as opposed to only at the

end of the cycle (as is the case in many reporting programs currently, wherein data is only shared at the end of the reporting cycle, after it is too late to make the appropriate adjustments).

3. The use of information technology (IT) systems will be necessary to effectively measure outcomes. Paper processes are becoming much more burdensome, and this will only become truer as the amount of data that must be collected and analyzed increases, which will likely be the case under an ACO model. Use of IT systems will likely be the only method by which providers and health organizations will be able to effectively capture the appropriate data and turn that data into useful, relevant information. Although an EHR will be one form of technology that is necessary, other quality reporting IT systems may also be needed to gather and report on the established metrics.

Patient Compliance

Compliance is viewed as the extent to which a person's behaviors coincide with medical advice.[5] Research indicates that noncompliance occurs in 50% to 75% of patients; this rate is even higher in patients with chronic illnesses or the elderly.[6] Patient compliance is a critical issue, not only because of its cost (which is estimated at as much as $100 billion per year),[7] but also its impact on patients, including hospitalization, development of complications, disease progression, premature disability, or death.[8] Both the cost associated with noncompliance and the diminished patient outcomes will be pivotal points to address under an ACO model, because both are metrics that are measured within the ACO structure.

Because compliance will play a significant role within an ACO, it will be incumbent on providers to take action to increase their own patients' level of compliance. The first step to increasing compliance will be to understand the reasons for noncompliance. These typically include the following:

- Misunderstanding prescribing or care instructions

- Denial/embarrassment

- Forgetfulness

- No faith in drug's effectiveness

- Reduction, fluctuation, or disappearance of symptoms

- Difficulty swallowing tablets or capsules

- Difficulty opening packages

- Adverse events

- Complex regimens

- Cost to patient

- Inconvenient or restrictive precautions[9]

Recognizing why people are typically noncompliant will help the provider tailor instructions and practices to best meet the needs of individual patients, thereby helping to increase compliance.

The second step that must be followed to help increase patient compliance is to implement a wide range of customization practices for each patient. Achieving optimal compliance involves a process of:

- Medication selection

- Choice of initial dose, dose interval, and subsequent adjustments

- Assessment of outcome

- Use of information from the patient and family or other caregiver

- Reexamination of the need for medications

- The attempt to avoid clinically significant drug-disease and drug-drug interactions[10]

When clinical care is individualized, it helps to ensure the process works for each patient; this will help increase compliance. In addition, this provision of patient-centered care is in keeping with one of the primary goals of an ACO model.

The third step for increasing patient compliance is communication with patients regarding expectations. One of the CMS requirements is that communications must be clear and easily understandable by beneficiaries. Providers must also improve the frequency of their communications, which includes follow-up with the patient when they are home. Many of the private and pilot ACOs established in 2010 and 2011 engaged a care coordinator to help improve communications and patient compliance. CMS is not going to bend a quality requirement if an ACO appeals and says that the patients were noncompliant and failed to follow instructions. It is the responsibility of the participating providers to deliver and follow-through on quality care, which means monitor the patient at home to ensure compliance. Providers will need to complete the following to help increase compliance with their patients:

- Express their (the provider's) perception that the medication/therapy/ follow-up appointment/etc. is important

- Provide clear and detailed instructions

- Create a drug regimen that fits the patient's schedule

- Explain the importance of compliance to the patient (and caregiver, if applicable)

- Instruct patients on how to self-monitor

- Contact/communicate with the patient *regularly*

- Provide written and visual aids to the patients (e.g., pamphlets, brochures, video education materials)

- Ask the patient to buy and use a medication container

- Ensure the patient completely understands what he or she must do at home to improve his or her healing process

- Ask the patient to repeat the instructions to the provider to confirm comprehension[11]

Note that increasing patient compliance should not be the sole responsibility of the provider. Rather, ACO groups may choose to use a patient care coordinator who is tasked with following up with patients, reminding them of their care instructions and the actions that need to be taken by the patient themselves.

Patient support structure—family and friends

Facing a serious medical condition can be a scary proposition for a patient, especially for the elderly; thus, many patients choose to lean on their family, friends, peers, and fellow patients for support. These support structures are valuable because they can help coordinate patient care, manage appointment scheduling, and increase patient compliance. Provider groups (on both the physician and hospital/health system level) can buoy the support provided by family and friends by taking the following actions:

- Create an online support group for both patients and patient supporters.

- Provide family and friends of current patients with the contact information of survivors and survivor supporters. (**Note:** Clearly, appropriate releases would need to be completed prior to divulgence of any contact information for former or current patients or patient supporters.)

- Staff a telephone support line that supporters can call to discuss pros and cons of treatment-related decisions.

- Offer seminars/workshops to educate patient supporters regarding disease-specific care and how they can best provide support to patients.

- Refer patients and patient supporters to appropriate mental health professionals who can help patients and supporters manage the psychological effects of illness.

- Patient supporters can serve a valuable function by assisting in patient care and ensuring that patients take appropriate steps to further their own care. The role of patient supporters will be another component to ensuring better quality outcomes under an ACO model.

Summary

ACOs have the potential to be the driver for quality that many within the healthcare industry have been searching for over the last decade and beyond. CMS believes the 33 quality measures identified in their SSP will help providers deliver improved quality of care to Medicare beneficiaries. Providers will need to be prepared to practice evidence-based medicine and to substantiate the care they provide with measurable outcomes. To help improve outcomes, providers will need to work to increase patient compliance with medical advice. In addition, providers will need to leverage patient supporters, such as family, friends, peers, and fellow patients, as part of the overall circle of caring that must exist. Going forward, quality must lie at the center of providers' clinical decision-making and the manner in which they treat their patients.

REFERENCES

1. Institute of Medicine. Crossing the Quality Chasm: A New Health System for the 21st Century. Washington DC: National Academy Press, 2001.

2. Shortell SM, Rundall TG, and Hsu J. *Improving Patient Care by Linking Evidence-Based Medicine and Evidence-Based Management.* Revised on June 12, 2007. *www.evidence-basedmanagement.org/ research_practice/articles/shortell_rundall_hsu_jama_2007.pdf* Accessed February 14, 2011.

3. Guidelines for Use of Medical Protocols," Connecticut Board of Examiners, February 4, 2004. *www.ct.gov/dph/lib/dph/phho/nursing_board/guidelines/guidelinesforuseofmedicalprotocols.pdf.* Accessed February 14, 2011.

4. Ibid.

5. Vance JE. *A Guide to Patient Safety in the Medical Practice.* American Medical Association, 2008.

6. Wertheimer AI and Santella TM, "Medication Compliance Research: Still So Far to Go." *The Journal of Applied Research in Clinical and Experimental Therapeutics,* 3(3): 2003. *www.jarcet.com/articles/ Vol3Iss3/Wertheimer.htm.* Accessed February 14, 2011.

7. Ibid.

8. Ibid.

9. Lamb M. "Improving Patient Compliance in Clinical Trials: Smart Packages or Smart Design." Almac Group. *www.almacgroup.com/papers/Papers/Improving_Patient_Compliance_in_CTS.pdf.* Accessed February 14, 2011.

10. Vance JE. *A Guide to Patient Safety in the Medical Practice.* American Medical Association, 2008.

11. Wertheimer AI and Santella TM. "Medication Compliance Research: Still So Far to Go," *The Journal of Applied Research in Clinical and Experimental Therapeutics,* 3(3): 2003. *www.jarcet.com/articles/ Vol3Iss3/Wertheimer.htm.* Accessed February 14, 2011.

The Role of Information Technology

Simply put, many experts believe that without information technology (IT) at the forefront, accountable care organizations (ACO) would not be able to exist. To attain success as an ACO requires collaboration among providers who are focused on patient care and outcomes. Accordingly, data sharing and integration of clinical and financial data is critical, and not just from a repository perspective or from the standpoint of health information exchange. Data must be delivered at the point of care; it must be up to date and organized in a meaningful way to prove outcomes and cost reductions. Without the ability to share and exchange information at the point of care, achieving the objectives of an ACO would be extremely limited, if not impossible. Nonetheless, several technology challenges loom ahead for ACOs. Although the final regulations do not require providers to have electronic health records (EHR), as outlined in Chapter 10, use of an EHR is a quality measure with a double point value. Healthcare technology will be an essential component for the success of any ACO, private or aligned with the Centers for Medicare & Medicaid Services (CMS).

Technology Considerations

The following are questions that should be addressed before formation of an ACO begins. These are often critical decision points that the parties should address up front.

Who provides the technology?

The first question to answer is who will provide the technology. Likely, all stakeholders will already have their own technology. Will it be best to have the solutions coexist or to develop a single enterprise solution? Trying to bring together multiple solutions can be extremely difficult because of data conflict and challenges with data reconciliation. For example, let's say practice "A" has an EHR system with vendor XYZ, but the patient is being seen at another location within the ACO, which operates a different EHR. Each practice is maintaining a different database, and each will have a unique patient identification number. Normally, an interface could help share data, but there could be hundreds of locations of care within an ACO. In this scenario, exchanging information and determining who will own the responsibilities for the technology becomes much more difficult. Options for exchanging and sharing information within an ACO are discussed later in this chapter.

Who owns and pays for the technology?

Another question to answer is the economics of sharing and distributing cost of owning and managing the technology. Most ACOs will centralize the technology into a shared data center or use cloud-based technology to optimize the benefits and as a way to substantially lower cost. (**Note:** Cloud-based technology, also known as "software as a service" (SaaS), allows a user to subscribe to the technology over the Internet. On-premise data centers or servers are not required.)

Who supports it?

Supporting the technology within an ACO is a critical success factor; it cannot be assumed that the vendors will provide support. ACOs require unique use of technology, especially its data. Most vendors are not structured to provide ACO support unless the ACO has engaged a vendor/supplier who provides these types of services.

Who ensures data integrity and that patient privacy is protected?

When multiple stakeholders share or feed data into a single platform, there will be a significant increase in the need to monitor and protect data integrity and patient privacy. Most ACOs use an industry best-practice policy called "break the glass" to manage patient privacy. (**Note:** Users will be allowed to access restricted areas of a patient chart, but they must first "break the glass," which will trigger an audit. In turn, the audit will determine if the access was legitimate or if a breach has occurred.)

Who owns the data?

The immediate reaction to this question is always the same: "The patient owns the data." However, the answer is more complicated and difficult to define within an ACO. If there are multiple providers all contributing to a single record, it is not easy to determine who compiled what unless the system can tract these entries by users, which most can. The issue is extracting the data by user and/or converting it back to the owner without pulling data everyone else many have contributed. Compliance standards, such as the continuity of care record and the continuity of care document, are mandated as a way to standardize what data should be allowed to move across different locations of care and what is necessary to de-convert. However, the ownership questions should be addressed contractually, and it should be stated that data is to be shared and owned by the entire ACO, regardless of who creates it.

Who controls what, and who creates and enforces the policies?

This one is easier to say than to do. ACOs are structured to work together as a single organization of care, under a single governance structure. However, each participant (other than hospital-employed physicians) will still be affiliated with their practice or other healthcare provider. Having a representative from their organization on the governing board of the ACO will help their voices be heard regarding policies, etc., but that is not necessarily possible or required under the CMS rulings. It is possible that each provider practice and hospital within an ACO will maintain their existing EHR technology, and interfaces will be written to share information. Everyone must comply with the technology system usage policies, or there could be substantial consequences. Some may perceive this as a loss of control; however, to avoid threats, the system must be managed through standards and end-user policies.

What if a physician or group does not have an EHR? How will their data be shared? CMS will provide claims data to an ACO for final usage review and cost analysis. However, an ACO must proactively and timely review its internal costs, results, etc., in order to meet the cost benchmarks and quality goals. How can the data from non-electronic environments be collected, reported, and analyzed? These are questions that each ACO must address.

How would one reverse (take apart) an ACO from a technology perspective?

Another important question to consider is the method for dismantling an ACO, should it not work out. The IT system would likely require support while everyone transitions off, and there would need to be some oversight as to how the data was transferred back to the caregivers and stakeholders. A de-conversion file should be vetted upfront, and each of the participants should clearly understand how they enter and exit the ACO.

Current State of the Health Information Technology Market as It Relates to ACOs

The concept of collaborating, exchanging, and integrating technology among multiple caregivers/stakeholders has existed for years. In fact, some will argue that ACOs are just another form of managed care, such as capitation or risk-based plans, which relied heavily on the monitoring of data for the purpose of reducing cost and the use of unnecessary services. However, under the capitation reimbursement system, the payers seemed to be the only source for the data, and they dictated the per member per month reimbursement. Providers argued that patients requiring the most care were often encouraged to take these plans, thus creating an adverse mix of patients. ACOs will have a similar shared risk model, but there will be a greater emphasis on use of technology.

A lot of the questions surrounding how ACOs will leverage technology can be answered by examining similar healthcare technology alliances existing today and solutions available to facilitate such collaboration. Various health IT (HIT) solutions typically exist within an ACO, including, but not limited to:

- EHRs

- Financial management systems

- Enterprise clinical information systems (integrated performance management and EHR systems)

- Computerized physician order entry (CPOE)

- Laboratory information systems (LIS)

- Radiology information systems (RIS)

- Document imaging management systems

- Picture archiving and communication systems (PACS)

- Data analytics software

- Accounting and customer relationship management software

Many of the familiar HIT alliances today are driven out of the need to improve technology and/or the need to become clinically integrated or to reduce the cost of IT spending. Some of these alliances are now evolving into ACOs. The recent improvements in healthcare technology, specifically EHRs, have created opportunities for multiple stakeholders—including competitors—to collaborate. Many trends have developed around IT collaboration and affiliations over the last several years (see "Types of IT Affiliations").

Although each of these affiliations has unique features, they all have one thing in common: sharing or participating in a single data repository and the desire to distribute data to multiple caregivers/stakeholders.

Required functionality for an ACO

When forming an ACO, formalizing who will manage, own, and support the technology should be one of the first steps. Models for sharing technology can vary significantly; however, it is critical to understand who controls the data and how it is used as well as the terms and conditions of the affiliation. Also, there are critical system requirements necessary for an ACO that must exist, including Health Insurance Portability and Accountability Act of 1996 compliance. The following functionality should be expected within any ACO technology solutions:

- The ability to detect when duplicate tests are being ordered. A primary objective for an ACO is to reduce costs by eliminating duplicate testing. Most systems can record an order and result, but they cannot detect if the test results already exists. A single vendor solution can usually accomplish this by organizing all of the test results into a single view. ACOs, with many solutions coexisting, will have to figure out a way to search the database of all the systems before ordering the test, which would result in an extra step for the provider.

TYPES OF IT AFFILIATIONS

Regional health information organizations (RHIO)

RHIOs are most commonly multistakeholder organizations responsible for clinical integration and information exchange. Generally, these stakeholders are developing a RHIO to affect the safety, quality, and efficiency of healthcare as well as access to healthcare information. RHIOs are always regional- or state-adopted and typically include payers, hospitals, physicians, and local employers. It is common for a RHIO to adopt a single EHR as a central repository for collecting clinical data. Security and user profiles (rights to access information) are critical in the setup of any RHIO. Although RHIOs offer many benefits, few have been successful due to financial instability. Initially, most funding comes from grants, but thereafter the stakeholders must contribute financially. Without critical mass numbers of participants, the cost can become too much to bear long-term due to the technology infrastructure required to support a RHIO.

Health information exchange (HIE)

Similar to RHIOs, HIE is defined as the mobilization of healthcare information electronically across organizations within a region or community. Software commonly known as a "master patient/person index" (MPI) is always required for HIE to exist. Without getting too technical, MPI creates a common identifier to which all other databases map. This allows information to move across multiple locations of care and across multiple platforms. It also enables clinical information to be electronically moved between different healthcare organizations, assuming each healthcare system can build a trust between the data being exchanged. A "trust," as a technical term, is the ability to verify the integrity of the data being exchanged, hence the need for the MPI. A secondary use of HIE can be for the purposes of public health, clinical, biomedical, and consumer health informatics research as well as institution and provider quality assessment and improvement.

Community health records (CHR)

A CHR is an EHR shared among several provider/medical practices in a single community. Often, the CHR is provided by the hospital to both its employed and nonemployed

TYPES OF IT AFFILIATIONS (CONT.)

medical staff. CHRs grew in popularity after the relaxation of the Stark Laws. CHRs may or may not include a practice management system, however, if the hospital operates a management service organization (MSO).

Application service providers (ASP)

An ASP is basically a spin-off of a data center. However, with the widespread adoption of the Internet and the development of Web-enabled and Web-based applications, software can now be delivered economically from a central server over the Internet. In some cases, physicians or hospitals will create their own ASP or contract with an ASP to deliver the application among all the stakeholders. The requirements are generally an Internet connection and a personal computer. Payment for services is typically a two- to three-year subscription based on a per provider per month hosting fee. Although ASPs offer affordability, one must accept some loss of control and ownership. All data is also stored off-site. Many ASPs will also provide revenue cycle management services.

Management service organizations (MSO)

MSOs have been around for many years and generally exist to allow hospitals to provide services to their medical staff as an alternative to ownership of the practices. They provide a blend of contract management and practice management services designed to maximize the efficiency and productivity of physician practices. An MSO can also decrease overhead costs by providing IT services and IT systems such as practice management software or an EHR.

Joint ventures and mergers

One of the primary reasons for considering a joint venture or merger is the ability to consolidate expenses and to share overheard. Joint vendors can entail a myriad of configurations that may or may not include a common IT infrastructure; however, in the case of a merger, consolidation of the IT systems is typical. Conversion and

TYPES OF IT AFFILIATIONS (CONT.)

transition planning is the greatest challenge. Mergers are similar to people who get married after living on their own for a while and end up with two of everything. All of the duplicate IT systems, specifically the practice management software and EHR software, must be consolidated into a single system. There must also be a strategy to retire the legacy systems and to complete data conversions. As medical practices become automated clinically, merging three or four disjointed EHRs into a single solution will become a challenge. Most physicians are very reluctant to give up an EHR that is working well, especially to move to one that they believe is inferior.

Software as a service (SaaS)

SaaS, also known as cloud computing, is becoming popular among ACOs because it allows for widespread distribution of data without the need for any single entity or stakeholder to manage the infrastructure or data center. Under a SaaS environment, the stakeholders would not own technology; users of the technology subscribe to it much as if it were a utility service. This removes a lot of the political issues because no one entity would own the system or be responsible for supporting the other stakeholders.

Source: Adapted from Physician Entrepreneurs: Strength in Numbers, *HCPro, 2008.*

- The ability to reconcile patient medications among all prescribers as a way to avoid waste and to avert drug-to-drug interactions. Drug-to-drug interaction is a major contributor to rising healthcare costs. Any system considered by an ACO must have the ability to reconcile medications across multiple caregivers and repositories.

- The system must have the ability to alert caregivers to the most cost-effective clinical guidelines without compromising patient care.

The Healthcare Executive's Guide to ACO Strategy

Decision support tools, alerts, and clinical guidelines are needed to drive compliance and outcome. Decision support tools are needed to provide feedback to the provider on the most cost-effective care based on clinical guidelines. These tools also encourage preventive maintenance and education tools for self-care for chronic problems.

- The ability to perform comprehensive analytics and data mining to evaluate outcomes, the ability to perform comprehensive analysis of data to evaluate patient care, and the effectiveness of the treatment are critical to the success of an ACO. It is essential for each ACO to track quality measures, costs, patient satisfaction, and so forth to meet the reporting requirements for CMS.

- Monitoring tools to incentivize behavior changes, such as evaluating usage and spending in contrast to outcomes. These tools will help with the management of the ACO and help drive the desired performance outcomes.

- Patient portal to communicate electronically in order to interact with patients in a safe and secure manner. A significant expectation of any ACO is to engage the patient and/or his or her family/caregivers and involve them in the healthcare (specifically, to hold them accountable for following orders and standards of care). Patient portal tools will allow for the patient and provider to share and exchange information securely and provide the patients with up-to-date information about their treatment.

Cost of sharing technology

As noted, an ACO must determine how the cost of sharing technology will be distributed among the stakeholders. Accordingly, there will be an upfront financial arrangement to acquire and procure technology solutions and services. An easy assumption is to distribute costs evenly, but what about special requirements and unforeseen circumstances? For example, what if one location of care requires the use of digital radiology and desires to purchase a PACS? Is the cost of the PACS distributed to all stakeholders or only those who benefit the most? If the PACS is used to store and distribute images for all providers, there may be the justification to spread the cost to everyone. To avoid circumstances such as these, the cost sharing method of choice is generally to assess a monthly hosting fee, although up-front payment may be required. The hosting fee is sometimes determined by distributing the cost among all the stakeholders; it can entail some remarkable economies of scale with greater numbers of participants.

If an entity establishes a goal to create and develop one shared system via the ACO, terms and conditions must be established for the members (see Figure 11.1). If the interest is to join or participate in an existing system, perhaps one owned by the hospital, knowing what terms to require of the members will be essential. The CMS guidelines require ACOs to form a legal structure within the laws of the state in which it operates and, of course, follow the CMS regulations. However, there is latitude regarding the participant composition. Under an ACO, there are likely two perspectives on affiliation:

1.   As a stakeholder/owner of the ACO or cofounder

2.   As a member or participating as a caregiver

FIGURE 11.1

MEMBERSHIP TERMS FROM BOTH PERSPECTIVES

TERMS FOR OWNERS DEVELOPING AN ALLIANCE	TERMS FOR MEMBERS PARTICIPATING
Must require members to pay a set-up fee.	Must get a guaranteed amount not to exceed and create payment terms based on project deliverable.
Must require members to pay a recurring hosting fee.	Establish a term that prevents the alliance from increasing the hosting fee without notice and/or that exceeds the consumer price index.
Must establish terms to charge for out-of-scope services.	Unauthorized services will not be covered expenses.
Must develop a user-acceptance policy; specifically, this should restrict software modifications and unauthorized access.	Ask to see the user-acceptance policy in advance. There may be some restrictions, especially with customization and modifications. Consider any access restrictions, especially from other hospitals.
Must create policies and procedures, including user manuals.	Restrict unauthorized use of your data and make sure liabilities are understood, especially if sharing a common medical record.
Must have the ability to monitor and audit.	Require some notice prior to being audited.
Updates and new releases should require some terms for acceptance and associated fees.	Require some testing before accepting updates. All updates should be included in the annual hosting fee.

FIGURE 11.1

MEMBERSHIP TERMS FROM BOTH PERSPECTIVES (CONT.)

TERMS FOR OWNERS DEVELOPING AN ALLIANCE	TERMS FOR MEMBERS PARTICIPATING
May want to limit assignment or require a transfer fee.	Do not enter into a contract unless the alliance will sign over the rights to use the software or provide you with the ability to transfer your support over to the software developer. The developer is the company who owns the software and may operate under a different name. You should always find out who owns the software code. As with any transfer, there will be added expenses and the need to purchase your own server to run the system independent of the alliance.

Harmonizing the ACO Through Connectivity

Another issue to confront will be connectivity. In most cases, each ACO stakeholder will need to establish its own connectivity to the central servers or join a network pre-established on behalf of the members. Figure 11.2 is a simple technical illustration of how these affiliations become networked together.

An ACO may also engage a HIE vendor who would facilitate the sharing and exchanging of data among the caregivers. If an HIE is not used, the ACO will need to enlist some type of master patient index (MPI) solution so data can be mapped across multiple locations of care. Generally, the EHR vendor will recommend an MPI solution or may even have its own MPI built into its solutions.

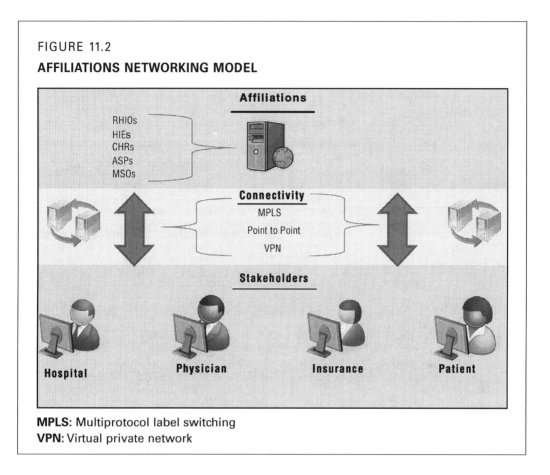

FIGURE 11.2

AFFILIATIONS NETWORKING MODEL

Affiliations

RHIOs
HIEs
CHRs
ASPs
MSOs

Connectivity

MPLS

Point to Point

VPN

Stakeholders

Hospital　　　**Physician**　　　**Insurance**　　　**Patient**

MPLS: Multiprotocol label switching
VPN: Virtual private network

This connectivity scenario will probably vary depending on the type of ACO, which is likely to fall into four different models:

1.　The multiple specialty group model. This model would likely be a single super group/private practice, with significant IT infrastructure already existing and the likelihood of an EHR already deployed. Under this model, the multiple specialty group would generally deploy on-premise servers and run its own data center out of its main location or in a hosting facility.

2. Independent provider association (IPA). Under this model, each location of care would likely have its own IT system and infrastructure, but they would all roll up to a single repository managed and supported by the IPA. Connectivity would likely be through a virtual private network or point-to-point dedicated data lines.

3. Physician-hospital organization. Typically, these stakeholders would jointly form an MSO that would act as the operations and management team for the ACO. The MSO would support the technology and many of the operational requirements, such as human resources, accounting, payroll, revenue cycle management, collections, etc.

4. Integrated health system. Under this model, the ACO likely would be formed using employed physicians and would operate completely under control of the hospital and use of the hospital's IT infrastructure and data center.

Summary

IT is critical to the success of an ACO. Access to patient data across all locations of care; medical management protocols, tools, and procedures for monitoring patient/provider adherence; contracting with health plans and employers; collection and distribution of dollars; and compliance with regulatory requirements at the state and federal levels requirements are all critical system requirements.

Quite frankly, every provider within an ACO must have electronic access if not a full EHR system in order to properly exchange data and report patient care. Any ACO being considered should consider the following:

- Examine existing infrastructure and solutions, obtain an in-depth understanding of what exists, and conduct a gap analysis to contrast what exists versus what is needed to accomplish the objectives of an ACO.

- Think through what the organization is looking to accomplish with its technology and define a strategic plan based on the model of choice, which could entail a single vendor enterprise approach, several solutions coexisting, or third-party HIE to bridge the gaps.

- Build an IT infrastructure to support the vision. Health IT purchases require forethought because there are nuances that are fulfilled by different vendors for different reasons. It is important to match the technology with the strategy defined in the second step.

- Allow plenty of time for planning and accept that a lot of uncertainty will exist. There will be the need to be flexible to adapt accordingly.

- Stick with the basics and do not over-engineer all your solutions when it comes to supporting new technology. A solid infrastructure and strong vendor partners are critical. Also build the infrastructure in a way that can adapt to future mandates and new policies.

The cost and effort associated with technology solutions and implementation are substantial. Therefore, having knowledgeable experts with relevant experience will be important to effectively implementing ACOs. In some cases, outsourcing to a third-party expert that is experienced in the development of ACOs may be necessary. Historically, assembling multiple stakeholders and agreeing on the options for sharing and distributing technology can get political and territorial. Having an objective, nonbiased third-party advisor can help alleviate these challenges. Stakeholders must accept that participating in any ACO will require increased willingness to accept substantial risk and some loss of control. However, the upside in compensation should be substantial and overhead should certainly be reduced, especially the spending on IT.

Patient-Centered Medical Homes

Today's multidimensional provision of healthcare, involving rising models such as accountable care organizations (ACO) and the patient-centered medical home (PCMH), can be traced to the past as an evolutional event. Focusing on the past, present, and future of the coordination of care, this chapter addresses how consolidation has shaped the future, discusses positioning in the evolving healthcare system, defines the PCMH, compares ACOs and medical homes, and projects where the future leads.

How Consolidation Has Shaped the Future

In 1998, Bruce Wasserstein, the now-deceased Wall Street investment banker widely recognized as one of the most notorious dealmakers since the Robber Baron era, wrote *Big Deal: 2000 and Beyond*,[1] which looked at some of the most significant trends and events driving corporate mergers and acquisitions over the last 50 years. In his section on healthcare mergers and acquisitions (M&A),

Wasserstein's assessment of the marketplace and his predictions for how health-care would look in the future were almost prophetic:

> *"The fundamental dilemma has become how to find more efficient means of production and delivery for healthcare while maintaining quality care. Structural innovation attempted to respond to these cost imperatives. Health maintenance organizations (HMOs), physician practice managers (PPMs), pharmacy benefit managers (PBMs), and managed care organizations have all cropped up in the last two decades. And for-profit hospitals have combined into empires to reduce costs. New players and innovative entrepreneurs have emerged to implement these new business models. Even the federal government's Medicare plan is not immune; Medicare providers will be subject to a prospective payment system (PPS) – akin to the system used by managed care companies in the private sector."*

In addition, Wasserstein described healthcare mergers as the result of trying to reduce the costs of healthcare. M&As provide organizations the opportunity to reduce cost by eliminating overhead and consolidating overlapping sales forces, Wasserstein explains. For example, he describes how a PPM model, in which individual physician practices would be bought and operated by PPM companies, would employ physicians and nurses, improve technology to better assess patient risks, and reduce costs by consolidating back-office functions and using the leverage with managed care companies provided by collective bargaining.

These views could have been written 20 days ago and have applied just as accurately as they did when Wasserstein first wrote them in the late 1990s. But his words were not prophetic in the sense that he made a prediction that later became reality. His assessment was meaningful because his analysis of the healthcare marketplace, looking at it from both a then and now viewpoint, illustrates how the trends driving the healthcare industry have been so cyclical to the point where any novice forecaster could make safe assessments as to what we should expect from the healthcare industry of the future.

The majority of players who have been around the healthcare industry for any amount of time have most likely lost count of how many times we have now come full circle in what seems like the most compelling example of a market as the hamster's wheel. As such, the difficult aspect of looking toward the healthcare industry of the future is not assessing what things will look like. The challenge is to identify how we can position ourselves to profit from knowing with reasonable probability what the future will bring. Perhaps it is not the same as Michael J. Fox's character Marty McFly's attempt to visit the future and bring back a sports almanac that would allow him to place guaranteed bets on sporting events. However, economists learn very early that the one thing that can both enhance market efficiency and eliminate it is access to information.[2]

How do we position ourselves to take advantage of opportunity when we have a good idea of what the future brings? The main thing we can do is look for the key trends that drove events in the past, measure the outcome of those events, and then determine where in the course of the events one benefited the most. Then, we can position ourselves strategically so that when history repeats itself, which we know the probability of it doing so is very high, we can make sure we are "in the right place at the right time."

Positioning for an Evolving Healthcare System

So what does all of this have to do with the healthcare industry today? One of the trends that everyone who spends any time within the healthcare industry has undoubtedly heard of is the emergence of the ACO. In looking back at Wasserstein's words, you could take any number of the acronyms he referred to, which were key drivers in the events that changed the healthcare industry during the '80s and '90s, and replace them with "ACO," and this would tell you a significant amount about where the healthcare industry is in the current evolution of the cycle.

Descriptions of ACOs by some physicians and healthcare executives may range from the industry's solution for the next model of healthcare delivery, to another form of capitation on steroids. And that does not include the standard cynicism of those who believe this is just another branch that the system will bounce off of as we continue plummeting off of the cliff.

ACOs have become the buzzword encompassing the broader trend of "clinical integration," which has been brewing for a number of years. The ACO model is being promoted as the solution for driving more coordination and thus, hopefully, quality in care between hospitals and physicians. At an operational level, how-ever, it really outlines the growing dynamic of formal affiliation between hospi-tals and physicians. But, of course, nothing will change something as big as our nation's healthcare system without plenty of conflict and challenges along the way, and the push for ACOs is no different.

In early January 2011, *The Washington Post* published a story on escalating conflict between groups representing physicians and managed care organizations centered on the financial structures that will be permitted under ACOs.[3]

> *[...] The ACO concept—like others in the health-care law that rejigger the financial relationships among providers and insurers—was written broadly. Lawmakers left it to regulators to figure out how to put the provisions into practice. The Centers for Medicare & Medicaid Services must flesh out many issues: Who can run an ACO? How are Medicare patients placed in ACOs and informed of these new arrangements? How is the caliber of care judged, and how will bonuses be awarded? What prevents these networks from becoming so large that they can dictate prices to private insurers?*

In my opinion, the question of what various ACOs will look like is less important at this point than the question of how they will change the current healthcare industry landscape. The most definite long-term impact we can expect is for this model to drive significant consolidation, as the clinical integration and physician alignment efforts that have developed thus far have already done so at significant levels. As such, we should not be surprised as we continue to watch hospitals, health systems, and physician groups come together through mergers, acquisitions, partnerships, and other affiliation models over the next 5–10 years.

Although many have already provided input as to what they think ACOs will look like and how they will impact the broader healthcare industry, it is important to consider those aspects of ACOs that are likely to give ACOs their true identity. Some of these different concepts and models that go hand-in-hand with the discussion of ACOs include physician-hospital alignment, integration, hospital M&A, and the PCMH. These concepts have multiple common traits; however, the one characteristic they all share—and share with ACOs—is the fact that the healthcare system is evolving toward an integrated model that provides scalable, streamlined solutions to healthcare consumers (i.e., patients) at the highest quality, as well as affordable and price-efficient financial structures to the suppliers and payers of these services.

What is the Patient-Centered Medical Home?

The PCMH or "medical home" model is one of those trends that encompass broader and quality care at more affordable and efficient pricing models. The medical home is as "an approach to providing comprehensive primary care that facilitates partnerships between individual patients, and their personal providers, and when appropriate, the patient's family."[4] The proposed benefit of the medical home concept is to expand access to healthcare for patients—including the insured and uninsured alike—and increase satisfaction of healthcare services through quality enhancements, thus resulting in an overall improvement of Americans' health.

The Patient Protection and Affordable Care Act requires the Secretary of the Department of Health and Human Services to establish grants for eligible entities who establish community-based interdisciplinary and inter-professional teams for primary care services. The ruling further says that these teams must support the PCMH, which is defined as a mode of care that encompasses:

1. Personal physicians

2. Whole-person orientation

3. Coordinated and integrated care

4. Safe and high-quality care through evidence-informed medicine, appropriate use of health information technology, and continuous quality improvements

5. Expanded access to care

6. Payment that recognizes added value from additional components of patient-centered care

According to Kevin Fickenscher, MD, former chief strategy and development officer at Dell Healthcare Services and founder and president of CREO Strategic Solutions, a healthcare consulting company, the key characteristics of a medical home include designation of a personal physician, care being coordinated around the patient's "whole needs," care coordination and integration, focus on evidence-based care and appropriately designated clinical outcomes, enhanced access to care, and a comprehensive payment model.[5] The overlying theme with these characteristics and the medical home model as a whole is that this concept is designed to provide a central and coordinated point of care for patients that is led by a primary care physician (PCP), but that is also streamlined to provide the highest quality of care throughout a patient's life, thus yielding the most optimal results.

The medical home concept is not a new idea that the industry has recently developed. Early discussions of this concept are traced to the late '60s, when a group of physicians affiliated with the American Academy of Pediatrics began to write about the need to offer more comprehensive healthcare over a patient's entire life. These physicians argued that if healthcare providers fail to take into consideration a patient's evolution of care, our system would likely migrate to a reactive healthcare delivery model, the result of which would be a general decline in the quality of patients' healthcare, due to the fact that providers would inevitably be too late in addressing critical needs.

This research was foretelling, in that this is exactly what has transpired within the healthcare delivery system in the United States over the past 30 years. This has resulted in a significant decline in the quality of healthcare, which in turn has resulted in two other downstream effects: (1) the cost of care has increased as the system has attempted to respond to quality issues, and (2) the access to care has declined due to both the quality and cost issues, making requirements for private health insurance more challenging. As such, the U.S. healthcare system can trace many of the challenges it faces today to the failure to consider a more comprehensive system of proactive medical care throughout a patient's life. Moreover, we can directly trace the effects of this failure to insurmountable costs in terms of economic costs and, more importantly, the cost of patients' lives.

Medical homes as a solution to solving challenges with declining healthcare quality have not completely been rejected by the industry since first being introduced. However, the concept is one that requires buy-in at the highest levels and then must be subsequently deployed throughout the system in order for it to really work. This is one of those concepts that is revolutionary in nature, based on where our system has evolved to over the past half-century, and as such, the system will require macro-level structural change in order for it to further evolve in the right direction. This level of widespread adoption throughout the industry just has not occurred; the primary reason for this has to do with the payment model that ultimately starts with the current state of the managed care and government reimbursement system. Again, we have come full circle with the evolution of continuous changes that the healthcare system seems to go through, as Wasserstein described more than a decade ago. Many times before that, other healthcare industry professionals pushed the medical home concept.

Seven key principles of the PCMH

According to the report, "Joint Principles of the Patient-Centered Medical Home," published in 2007 by the American Academy of Family Physicians, the American Academy of Pediatrics, the American College of Physicians, and the American Osteopathic Association, there are seven key principles of the PCMH.

1. Establishing an ongoing relationship

The first principle is that each patient should have an "ongoing relationship with a personal physician trained to provide first contact, continuous, and comprehensive care," the report says. This ongoing relationship should constitute consistent care over an extended time frame of a patient's life, perhaps a patient's entire life (obviously divided between adolescent and adult years). Further, this principle serves as the basis of the medical home concept, in that a patient's PCP should also serve as a point of contact for the patient's healthcare needs. This means that although the PCP should not attempt to extend his or her services beyond their appropriate boundaries, this provider can assist in coordinating a further range of comprehensive care as needed by the patient.

This concept, however, results in two additional assumptions. First, the PCPs will have greater responsibilities to their patients, perhaps even beyond the exam room encounter, which they must accept and be equipped to handle, in addition to being compensated for this additional responsibility. Second, the infrastructure and tools used by providers within the system must be enhanced so that PCPs can efficiently communicate and exchange information with specialists and other providers as needed throughout a patient's continuum of care.

2. Physician-directed care

The second principle addresses the need of a physician-directed medical practice, which according to the joint report means the personal physician "leads a team of individuals at the practice level who collectively take responsibility for the ongoing care of patients."

3. Taking a holistic view

The third principle is what the authors of the report referred to as "whole person orientation," which they described as a patient's personal physician being "responsible for providing all the patient's healthcare needs [and] taking responsibility for appropriately arranging care with other qualified professionals." These last two principles, in some ways, address the question of additional responsibility that PCPs will have to take on under this concept; however, much is left to interpretation as to how this model would actually be executed. Further, this concept assumes that such a model could just fall into place; however, we have learned from previously failed models that unless there is a corresponding payment or economic model that compensates providers for additional requirements, the chances of that model proving sustainable are slim.

4. Coordinating care across the continuum

Continuing on, the fourth principle states that a patient's care should be "coordinated and/or integrated, for example across specialists, hospitals, home health agencies, and nursing homes." This is that concept that illustrates how the medical home model will provide patients with a centralized point of contact for coordinating all healthcare needs throughout the patient's life. So when a patient needs back surgery, the role of the PCP is more of a coordinator between the neurosurgeon, orthopedists, pain management specialists and anesthesiologists, physical therapists, radiologists, hospital staff, and other providers that participate in this ongoing episode of patient care.

5. Focus on care planning

The fifth principle mentioned in the report attempts to bridge the concept of comprehensive care to enhanced quality for the patient. This principle states that quality and safety should be assured through a care planning process, as well as through the application of proven methodologies of evidence-based medicine, clinical decision support tools, performance measurement, active participation of patients in decision-making, information technology, a voluntary recognition process, quality improvement activities, and other measures. Although seemingly obvious on the surface, this is actually one of those areas that has proven to be most challenging for the providers to accept, the reason for which has nothing to do with them questioning their dedication to providing the utmost quality in care. The reason why concepts such as "clinical-based outcomes" often turn doctors off is because they know better than anyone that every patient and each encounter is different and inherently unique, and although there are standards that can and should be followed, attempting to apply all aspects of clinical management to outcomes would require the incorporation of too many variables and externalities that often simply cannot be controlled.

However, this does not mean performance measures and evidence-based medicine are altogether failing concepts. These and many other solutions adopted by physicians over the years have proven to change the approach that practitioners take to managing a patient's long-term health for the better. Moreover, as we continue to develop new models, tools, and technological resources allowing for the enhanced management of patient care, the result clearly has been a marked improvement in quality for patients over the long run.

6. Improved access to care

Enhanced access to care is the sixth principle from the report, and this speaks to the call for ACOs and medical homes to not only increase the availability of healthcare services to patients, but to simply make them more accessible so that there is never confusion for the patient as to whether or not he or she can receive critical care that is needed. According to the report, care can be more accessible through "open scheduling, expanded hours, and new options for communication."

The trend of medical groups evolving toward more nonconventional patient communication techniques and hours of operations shows that patients' needs and expectations of their healthcare providers are becoming more integrated in that they are demanding similar levels of care and response from their physicians' practice that they would expect to receive from a hospital or other facility. This is a key area where the medical home concept will be critical to the growth of ACOs because as they operate today, most medical practices are not fully equipped to meet all of the needs and expectations of their patients when it comes to these more nontraditional services. Technology is a critical aspect of these services, allowing physicians and other clinicians to communicate in new ways with patients while also allowing patients to receive information and other remote services available outside the practice. However, not every practice can acquire the technology that allows these services to be available for patients. The medical home concept can bridge this higher level of service using some of those unconventional methods while continuing to allow for streamlined care for the patient at reasonable costs and time demands for the providers.

7. Reconciling payment with the value

Finally, the report's last and seventh principle is that payments to medical providers under the medical home model "must appropriately recognize the added value provided to patients." There is a distinct framework on which the report states payments for medical home services should be based, which includes the fact that payments should reflect the value of "work that falls outside of the face-to-face visit"; should "support adoption and use of health information technology for quality improvement"; and should "recognize case mix differences in the patient population being treated within the practice," among other key elements. Overall, it is critical that the clinicians providing services under the medical home model are justly compensated for their work; otherwise, the model will never be effective. This principle contributes to the broader tenant of the overall medical home concept, which says that in order for this model to be effective and in order for patients and the healthcare industry to realize value and long-term improvements from it, the key legs of the stool must all be firmly in place and adhered to; otherwise, we are going down another path that will surely lead to insufficient results.

Comparing ACOs and Medical Homes

Clearly, there are many similarities between ACOs and the medical home concept. Kevin Fickenscher, MD, commented on this in a 2011 article: "Rather than tackling payment reform in isolation of care delivery, [ACOs] and medical homes offer a consolidated approach to both issues."[6] Fickenscher argues that ACOs and medical homes are also similar in that both "consolidate multiple levels of care for patients." This means that both models are intended to increase the level of access to care for patients while at the same time making that care process more efficient and delivered at a higher quality.

In the same way that there are many synergies between the ACOs and medical homes, there are also some key differences. Fickenscher argues that whereas medical homes are structured such that the PCP serves as the hub of the clinical care team, ACOs focus on coordinating multiple segments and sources of care for a patient in a centralized fashion.[7] Although this difference may seem like a technicality to some, it is critical when considering a medical provider's approach to care because many providers will argue that one approach over the other could make a significant difference in the quality of care that patients receive.

The medical home model, in some ways, is analogous to the hospitalist model in an acute and/or emergent care situation, where a single physician can serve as the central point for coordinating and facilitating patient care throughout the time that patient stays within the hospital's walls. However, that care will typically end once the patient is discharged (though not always). Indeed, many hospitalists have for years been extending their services to patients far beyond their initial hospital encounter, and in many cases, this includes coordinating care for them with specialists and other specific needs. Likewise, the medical home focuses on centralizing that care process even further, such that the PCP would coordinate all of that care, perhaps even prior to encountering a hospitalist within an acute or emergent care situation if the urgency of a case allowed such coordination.

ACOs, on the other hand, address a higher level of organization and infrastructure across the care continuum. This focuses more on the idea of developing a single system or series of facilities that can provide practically all elements of care in a much more centralized or vertically integrated manner. ACOs comprise integrated organizations of care, including primary care, acute care, and specialized care. And the value proposition is that an integrated care delivery team can provide better results when coordinating care for a patient, as opposed to the silo effect that has been directly linked to causing many negative health effects for patients and costs the healthcare system billions of dollars every year. Integrating those resources in efforts to better coordinate care allows for that PCP in the medical home to more efficiently manage the patient's care within a system that has all of the resources needed essentially in a one-stop-shop fashion.

Healthcare executives and physicians have been observing the successes and failures of the many attempts over the last few decades to implement strategies similar to ACOs and medical homes. But, as the industry begins to learn more about these new models, which are really just evolved and improved-on versions of older concepts, many participants of the industry are beginning to see the potential value that could come from them. However, the aspect of the discussions today that is becoming clear to those who are closely observing these new trends is that many, if not most, of these ideas being proposed are very good.

The medical home concept is clearly innovative and well-considered; the positive impact on both patients and providers could truly be significant. Even though the ACO and medical home concepts are still being refined and developed, the question is not whether these are good ideas or bad ideas. Improving healthcare is at the core of this entire discussion, and though various groups and individuals may differ in their opinions as to what concept will work better than others, the concern that most industry stakeholders are considering now is whether we will be able to adequately execute any of these models.

Summary

Whoever said "wins are 90% preparation and 10% execution" most likely did not work within the U.S. healthcare industry, because one thing we have never lacked is ideas, nor have we ever shied away from spending money on preparation, which is a key component to the success of any new program or initiative. But neither preparation nor execution means anything unless that preparation is sufficient to allow for effective execution. And even if we provide the greatest preparation imaginable, it will mean nothing if the industry and regulators cannot work together to execute these models effectively and efficiently.

REFERENCES

1. Wasserstein, Bruce, *Big Deal: 2000 and Beyond.* New York: Warner, 1998, p 481–484.

2. *Back to the Future®.* Universal Studios, 1985.

3. Rau, Jordan, "Insurers, health-care providers at odds on rules for 'accountable care organizations." *The Washington Post*, January 2011. *www.washingtonpost.com/wp-dyn/content/article/2011/01/09/AR2011010903401.html.* Accessed March 4, 2011.

4. American Academy of Family Physicians, American Academy of Pediatrics, American College of Physicians, and American Osteopathic Association. "Joint principles of the patient-centered medical home." 2007. *www.pcpcc.net/content/joint-principles-patient-centered-medical-home.* Accessed March 4, 2011.

5. Fickenscher, Kevin MD. "Accountable Care Organization (ACO) and Medical Home Differences." MedPage Today: KevinMD.com, January 2011. *www.kevinmd.com/blog/2011/01/top-stories-health-medicine-morning-january-8-2011.html.* Accessed March 4, 2011.

6. Fickenscher, ibid.

7. Fickenscher, ibid.

Where Do We Go From Here?

Whether you are reading this book as a physician leader in your own practice or as a physician or hospital executive, you are probably considering what steps to take next. This conclusion recaps the major requirements for moving into ACOs, as discussed more thoroughly in prior chapters, including the requirements for a new way of thinking about delivery of healthcare.

Physicians and Hospitals Need to Form Alliances

As outlined in Chapter 4, there is much to be gained when hospitals and physicians choose to work together. It no longer makes sense for physicians to mistrust or compete with hospitals due to reimbursement trends. The overall economics of private practice are clearly pushing the two closer together. Major challenges associated with pursuing an alignment model can include the following:

- Operational

- Autonomy and control

- Trust

- Competition

- Sharing revenue

However, many are able to overcome these challenges and realize true success. What is exciting is there are so many ways that hospitals and physicians can partner. Following are various alignment alternatives for hospitals and physicians, as detailed in Chapter 4:

- Limited alignment arrangements

    - Managed care networks

    - Call coverage stipends

    - Medical directorships

    - Recruitment guarantees

- Moderate alignment initiatives

    - Management services organizations

    - Targeted cost incentives

    - Joint ventures

    - Clinical co-management/service line management

- Full alignment

  – Clinic model

  – Employment

  – Professional services agreement for comprehensive professional services

Both hospitals and physicians should take a step back and assess what their long term vision is for one, three, and five years into the future. Then, they should begin to consider how they can achieve that vision through the previously stated models. As alignment evolves, other models (or hybrids of existing ones) will develop, especially as ACOs become more common, even in the private sector of payer/provider relationships. What is great about alignment is that some form of integration can be achieved by practically all physicians and hospitals. Whereas some may choose, and rightfully so, that a limited alignment model is best for them, others may directly pursue full alignment. Often, once an initial alignment occurs, the parties develop trust, mutual respect, and a common sense of purpose that leads to an even stronger affiliation down the road. Even combinations of the various models often result.

Undoubtedly, we expect the healthcare industry to look very different in years to come. While ACOs and other initiatives will continue to change the reimbursement landscape, various forms of alignment will transform the hospital/physician landscape as both attempt to respond to the changing reimbursement. For sure, we work and operate in a dynamic industry and as such, structures and relationships vary and adjust over the years. With or without ACOs (or something comparable), this characteristic is likely to continue.

Attitude Adjustment: Partnering in the Delivery of Quality and Cost-Effective Medical Care

The healthcare industry has seen plenty of change over the past 50 years. Yesterday's healthcare business model focused on the providers, (individual) productivity was the primary dynamic, and price was the driving factor. Tomorrow's models must be more patient-centered with the focus on quality-based outcomes. The real focus will be on preventing illnesses or reoccurrences, reducing hospitalizations, and thus reducing costs. Although volume will continue to be important, it will be couched within a different setting—one focused on efficiency and information sharing—not merely numbers of encounters and procedures.

Highly motivated and dedicated individuals who can work as a team will be required to achieve a successful ACO or some other new entity similar to an ACO. America produces the most skilled and knowledgeable physicians in the world, but this type of expertise must be supplemented with other skills to get us on our next journey to improved healthcare of our communities. Medical providers will need to modify their behavior and be managers of change. They will need to learn to re-tool their treatment patterns to achieve quality outcomes, while maintaining an appropriate level of productivity. The provider of tomorrow must truly partner with the other providers to bring synergy and shared results to the patients and ACO entity. They can no longer view themselves individually; they must understand their role as an integral member of a special team with common goals and objectives. Results can only be achieved through coordinated teamwork. Remember, there is no "I" in "team." Egos will need to be checked at the door so that the new team culture can emerge.

The new attitudes will underscore the patient-centered focus for quality outcomes and improved health for the chronically ill. Team attitudes are essential and will help bond medical professionals and remind them of the real reason they chose medicine as their career path—to prevent illness when possible and to treat sick patients in the most effective manner.

Review Current Compensation and Reimbursement Models and Plans

As we discussed at length in Chapter 5, the introduction of ACOs, as well as other forms of outcomes-based reimbursement, will have a significant role in shaping compensation and reimbursement models of the future. The change to reimbursement models is inevitable because that is at the heart of the ACO process; moving from use-based to value-based reimbursement structures. Clearly, this can and will take many different forms, the least of which are outlined here:

- Fee-for-service (at least the continuation of some form of such)

- Bundled payments

- Medical home payments

- Capitation

- Blended payments

- Incentive/risk sharing

With regard to reimbursement models, some changes relative to such will be forced by Medicare and other payers, while others will be voluntary. Similar to many other Medicare programs, ACOs will likely become more "forced" over time. Meaning, at first, organizations will have an opportunity to join, with potential for incentives; in the future; however, it is likely that organizations will be required to participate and penalized if they do not. Although the enforcement may not be for several years (if ever, should ACOs prove not to be effective or adopted in the private sector), most organizations would be best served to begin taking some action relative to pursuing new reimbursement alternatives. The following two steps should be considered by these organizations:

1. Assess current infrastructure capabilities, including physician alignment and technology infrastructure. As discussed throughout this book, these two components will be critical to organizations, especially hospitals, pursuing value-based reimbursement arrangements. Thus, without a solid information technology (IT) infrastructure in place and good alignment with physicians, the success in a value-based reimbursement model will be limited at best. If an organization is not moving ahead in these areas, it should become a top priority that is factored into its strategic plan. At a minimum, providers should prepare for accountable care by assuring that their IT infrastructure is solid for now and the future.

2. Consider core competences relative to quality and other value-based areas and pursue those. Once an organization has a solid infrastructure (both from a physician personnel and technology standpoint), they

should begin to assess their strengths in terms of quality, patient satisfaction, cost control, etc. This should occur on a service line basis. Where there is already success or some room for relatively easy improvement, those areas should be pursued with third-party payers for potential reimbursement incentives. Further, this process will lay the foundation for the organization's potential success within an ACO structure.

As outlined earlier in the book, the push toward ACOs is clearly leading to an increase in physician employment by health systems in order to ensure that the needed physicians are available to support an ACO and other new reimbursement paradigms. With this comes the need to compensate the physicians, in most cases under an incentive-based arrangement.

Historically, due to the reimbursement structures in place, these incentive models have largely been focused on productivity, using charges, collections, or work relative value units (wRVU). The onset of ACO-type structures is pushing toward a greater emphasis on non-productivity related criteria. We anticipate that this trend will continue as the reimbursement paradigm shifts. Specifically, where quality incentives may have represented 2%–10% of pay in the past, they may represent 15%–40% in the future.

Although non-productivity incentives are becoming more commonplace, some level of productivity must still be required. As an extreme example, it is not viable for a physician to only take care of one patient per day really well. Although quality would likely be excellent, there would be no money to pay the bills. What we believe is most likely to occur is an overlap of productivity and non-productivity incentives. In essence, to earn incentive pay, the physician would not only be required to achieve a minimum standard of productivity, but would also be required to achieve certain quality and patient satisfaction measures. Thus, the physician must earn the incentive once by simply doing the work required and a second time by performing the work in such a way to meet the non-productivity objectives. This will shift more risk to the physician, but it will likely occur gradually only as reimbursement moves in this direction.

For hospitals that currently employ physicians, it is important to start reassessing the existing compensation models and, at a minimum, ensuring that there is some focus other than on productivity. Similarly, this is difficult to achieve without proper technology systems in place to capture non-productivity data. It is impossible to compensate a physician on factors that require data unless it is being tracked. Further, in terms of long-term thinking, it may make sense to begin considering how the productivity and non-productivity incentives can be blended together. The key is to ensure that the risk and reward are properly balanced for both the physician and health system.

Recap of the ACO Programs

The philosophy of the ACO concept to focus on the patient for his or her self-involvement, to improve customer service, to improve care at an individual and community level, and to reduce costs without adversely affecting quality are not new to many providers and is not at all foreign to the entire healthcare industry. Some are practicing several of these goals already. Those who are not mostly understand and appreciate the need to do so. What makes the ACO concept so unique is the unity of separate providers under one large umbrella (i.e., the ACO entity) to coordinate the care of certain patients while still remaining "separate" as provider units, yet sharing in savings (and possibly losses) as a group. This will require a very different culture and a willingness to put egos on the shelf and work in harmony at all times for the best interest of the patients and the ACO. Further, it shifts the previous emphasis that economically encouraged high utilization and testing to consideration of the patient care holistically, as with the patient-centered medical home (PCMH).

As we have outlined previously, ACOs can be managed by the private sector or organized under the CMS program. Numerous private ACOs exist at the time of this publication. Each provider will need to decide whether to participate in any type of ACO; and if the decision is to move in that direction, then the next decision is a private entity or CMS model.

The table below represents a regulatory impact analysis included by HHS in the final regulations document released in October 2011. It outlines their best estimate of the costs and benefits of the SSP. The dollars are estimates by CMS based upon their projected participation in the ACO program. These estimates are questionable since the number of CMS ACOs to be formed for the first contract period of 2012 through 2015 is unknown.

FIGURE A

ESTIMATED NET FEDERAL SAVINGS, COSTS AND BENEFITS CYs 2012–2015

	CY 2012	CY 2013	CY 2014	CY 2015	CYs (2012–2015)
Net federal savings					
10th percentile	-$30 million	-$20 million	$10 million	$0 million	$0 million
Median	$20 million	$90 million	$160 million	$190 million	$470 million
90th percentile	$70 million	$210 million	$320 million	$370 million	$940 million
ACO bonus payments					
10th percentile	$60 million	$180 million	$280 million	$360 million	$890 million
Median	$100 million	$280 million	$410 million	$520 million	$1,310 million
90th percentile	$170 million	$420 million	$600 million	$740 million	$1,900 million
Costs	The estimated startup investment costs for participating ACOs range from $29 million to $157 million, with annual ongoing costs ranging from $63 million to $342 million, for the anticipated range of 50–270 participating ACOs. With the mean participation of ACOs, the estimated aggregate start-up investment and four-year operation costs is $451 million.				
Benefits	Improved healthcare delivery and quality of care and better communication to beneficiaries through patient-centered care.				

*Note that the percentiles for each individual year do not necessarily sum to equal the percentiles estimated for the total four-year impact, in the column labeled CYs 2012–2015, due to annual and overall distributions being constructed independently.

Source: U.S. Department of Health and Human Services, Centers for Medicare & Medicaid Services. Medicare Program: Medicare Shared Savings Program: Accountable Care Organizations. Fed Reg. 2011–27461; 42 CFR Part 425; [CMS-1345-F] RIN 0938-AQ22, 593.

Key points for review

We have covered a lot of information in this book regarding the ACO concept with a specific emphasis on the CMS SSP. Although there are numerous pilots actively in progress for accountable care (see Appendix A for an overview) and a few with the PCMH model, most have not been in existence long enough to sufficiently determine the overall results of their program as well as the return on investment. There is little doubt that our healthcare system needs to be improved, both financially and in patient quality. How we get there is a journey still to be determined. The following summarizes some of the key elements we have presented in the previous chapters.

Physician-hospital alignment is the key ingredient for a successful ACO entity. Physicians, hospitals, and other providers must align with each other to ensure a common vision and goals. Under the CMS SSP, they will continue to function and bill as separate organizations; however, they must become one united group for the coordinated patient care, improved quality, and reduction of claim dollars. Key participants of some of the ACO pilots have said the greatest challenge they faced was the new culture required under the new entity. Some of them voiced their opinion that it could take a group several years to adopt the "right" culture to succeed as an ACO.

Legal considerations will be a greater challenge for private ACOs because they are not receiving some of the waivers or special considerations that groups will receive from the Federal Trade Commission, the Department of Justice, and the Office of Inspector General for a CMS ACO. All parties need to be cognizant of the antitrust and anti-kickback laws and ensure they are not in violation.

A readiness assessment is an important step to take if you are considering an ACO alignment. This would include organizational and IT assessments, review of the leadership team and culture, market analysis, and an assessment of current alignments (physician-to-physician and physician-to-hospital). A financial review would also be beneficial because there will be startup and ongoing management costs. This type of assessment will assist an organization in making a decision to move forward with an ACO, make needed changes required to move to an ACO environment in the future, or simply remain under current structure.

Benchmarks for cost goals need to be established whether a private or CMS entity is formed. The United States has the highest per capita healthcare cost of all developed countries in the world, yet we are not rated as the number one provider of quality healthcare by the World Health Organization. HHS has detailed how cost benchmarks will be established for the SSP using claim history and adjusting for trends and certain risk factors for the assigned beneficiaries. The beneficiary assignments will be reviewed quarterly and benchmarks will be adjusted annually.

Quality measures have been an important measurement in healthcare for years. PQRS was first implemented in 2007 (as PQRI) and continues today to measure and reward for quality. There are other quality programs also active today. Many of the private ACOs are focusing only on some of the key chronic conditions, such as diabetes and heart disease. Although costs are important, their thrust is truly on quality and improving the lives of these patients living with moderate to severe chronic conditions. Evidence-based medicine is a critical component of the CMS ACO program and protocols will be used to attain goals.

IT is another critical element in any successful accountable care organization. Electronic health records and a robust, stable IT infrastructure will be essential to record, share, report, and analyze data—both quality and cost. Without the ability to electronically share and analyze data, an ACO will be handicapped in how it can "move" paper data from provider to provider in an extremely timely manner.

PCMHs are also becoming the new age of ambulatory care and will grow whether or not aligned with any type of ACO. It is anticipated the PCMHs will play a significant role in the care of our aging baby boomer generation. The focus is to better improve care, concentrate on the patient's involvement of their care, reduce inpatient and emergency room admissions, and help patients lead a better life outside of an institution. We believe that a successful ACO will include a PCMH within its treatment structure.

The CMS SSP is the government's tool to improve the quality of patient care while reducing expenses and offering a monetary incentive to providers. CMS will assign Medicare beneficiaries from the fee-for-service program into an ACO based upon their primary care provider's participation in an ACO entity. There are two models within the SSP and the shared savings rates vary by model and level of success. If quality measures and cost benchmarks are met, ACOs will be eligible to receive savings to share among the participating providers. If a certain level of loss is incurred under the Track 2 model, the ACO will be required to repay the losses to CMS.

Change is inevitable, and the healthcare industry has experienced plenty of it. Change will continue into our future and the generations after us; we cannot imagine what changes will take shape into the vast future. Managed care of the 1980s undoubtedly changed the way providers practiced medicine and delivered healthcare. Physician-hospital integration has also contributed to new alliances and trends that have improved relationships, changed compensation models, and modified the lifestyles of participating physicians. Continuing pressures to increase productivity, coupled with reduced reimbursements from both private payers and CMS, have greatly challenged all medical professionals, both the hospital and physician sectors. All of these changes and pressures have illustrated certain characteristics of the American healthcare providers—flexibility and the ability to adopt to change. Whatever the next stage is with ACOs and beyond, continued change and adaptation will be required.

Pilot Programs

Health systems, hospitals and physician groups launched numerous pilots for ACO pilots throughout the country following the signing of the Patient Protection and Affordable Care Act (PPACA) in March 2010. All of the pilots are private models with healthcare providers forming entities based upon their perception of what an ACO should look like and what it needs to accomplish. They had an opportunity to choose their models as many began even before the proposed CMS regulations were issued in March of 2011. One of the most notable pilots is the Brookings-Dartmouth ACO Pilot Project. This organization is sponsoring five pilots in various locations.

This section discusses one of the Brookings-Dartmouth pilots (Norton) and a free-standing ACO pilot in New Hampshire. The information provided two pilots featured are by Norton Healthcare, Kentucky's largest healthcare system with more than 40 locations, and Dartmouth-Hitchcock Health Care System, a multi-facility healthcare system servicing New Hampshire. These two organizations have launched successful ACO pilot programs and are achieving the desired goals and objectives that most organizations would like to achieve. The information provided here by individuals in these organizations is shared willingly for readers of this book.

Review of the Norton Healthcare and Dartmouth-Hitchcock Health Care System ACOs

Pursuing the delivery of higher quality, improved safety, and increased patient satisfaction, Norton Healthcare determined that their ACO pilot project would be the most appropriate vehicle to achieve their goals. This project has provided Norton with a sense of urgency and focus around what they were ultimately trying to achieve.

Consolidation of Services

When it comes to consolidation of services in most hospital environments, there are many areas where improvement can be achieved. At present, Norton has approximately 400 employed physicians across approximately 80 access locations. Roughly half of their physicians are in primary care specialties. Based on the economics and market conditions, as well as the growing need for additional physicians, Norton anticipates this number will increase in the very near future.

Norton's organizational efforts and strategic mind-set has helped facilitate consolidation in diagnostic testing centers, bariatric surgery, and immediate care centers, which are typically located at the diagnostic centers. In order to achieve appropriate consolidation of services within the core scope of achieving quality outcomes objectives, it is important to recognize which areas an organization should begin to track and monitor as well as other areas for improvement in the future.

Norton's one area of strategic focus was the standardization of care processes across their organizational practices in how patients with particular diagnoses were managed. Examples of these would be to standardize the treatment proto-cols for lower back pain and patients with congestive heart failure.

Other areas of focus required fundamental clinic re-engineering at the ambula-tory level. Specifically, this included rates of generic prescribing; educating physi-cians and providers; and improving vaccination rates, systems of care, and cancer prevention screening care. By analyzing current practices and standardizing treatment care protocols within the organization, the systems will be able to focus on improving quality and patient satisfaction as well as cost management. As might be anticipated with any health system or organization, old habits die hard. For years, hospitals have created various silos within their own walls that lead to turf battles and distractions from achieving big picture goals and objec-tives. Examples of these areas that one might encounter include the following:

- Contracted services in hospital-based specialties

- Centers of excellence

- Internal physician cultures

- Diagnostic imaging

- Individual practice styles and location variances

- Supply chain protocols

- Group purchasing arrangements and even multiple hospitals within a common market

All have the potential to detract from or undermine the overall goals and objectives of the system unless they are managed and addressed appropriately.

Organizations that want to develop an ACO should establish and create strong physician leadership teams and work groups that help communicate the goals and objectives of the organization. As much as possible, the leadership must make every effort to ensure that all team members are on the same page. This does not mean there will never be discrepancies or varied opinions. In fact, it is quite the opposite. The goal is to create a structural format that manages consistent treatment protocols, ensuring high patient satisfaction with positive outcomes. The physician work groups and teams should encourage varying opinions to challenge whether they are providing the highest level of care for their patients/customers.

As health systems across the country race to create stronger, more diverse employed practice or affiliated physician alignment models, the occurrence of physicians coming together in similar specialties with diverse opinions and backgrounds increases substantially. Key surgical and medicine subspecialty areas such as orthopedics, spine, cardiology, and oncology must consider how they can best work together to accomplish these goals and objectives. Presently, this strategy occurs more frequently in metropolitan markets. However, groups in suburban and ultimately rural areas will also need to address similar medical staff and specialty cultural challenges. For disparate groups to be more cohesive, it is important to have these standardizations of processes and protocols established within a particular service line and organization.

Meshing of physician cultures and practice styles is one of the greatest challenges facing the development of a successful alignment model. In most cases, this takes time to accomplish and requires the merging parties to be willing to cooperate. It also calls for strong physician and administration leadership development. Therefore, it is important to bring all physicians within the organization under the same entity to achieve the scope and dynamics required for the system objectives.

Development of the desired culture was not difficult in the Dartmouth-Hitchcock organization because the physicians saw that a focus on quality outcomes and cost management was the right thing to do. Although it is hard to argue with doing what is right, it is important to communicate the objective and to cast the overarching vision in a way that the organization understands the importance of achieving this goal. At that point, it becomes more about gaining consensus on how to achieve these goals rather than "should we or shouldn't we" pursue the goals.

Group Purchasing

Group purchasing plays an instrumental role in helping to achieve managed cost. To achieve the overall goals and objectives for the ACO, a strong clinical informatics system is imperative. Through the proper group purchasing and clinical informatics processes, organizations can try to streamline any opportunity that would allow improved quality while achieving various cost savings.

For Norton Healthcare's administration, this meant being more cognizant of the outcome of various physician preferences and their success factors. Unless a hospital administration manages these initiatives appropriately, this concept can create quite a negative stir among physicians. Norton's processes are based on the mind-set that, from an administrative perspective, physicians do not need to be told what they can or cannot use or how they should choose to practice medicine. The physicians are the clinicians; administration and group purchasing are not. As organizations evolve into more integrated models, they are more apt to breach physician autonomy.

Norton decided that they needed to find a way to discern whether a device would be acceptable for their organization. Thus, they formed a technology assessment committee where a physician panel looks at all physician requests for formulary additions or medical supplies that the physician or physicians prefer. Physicians who want to add items must follow a lengthy application process to substantiate why they want this particular item and what they believe it will achieve and accomplish for their patients. In addition, physicians must then present the request to the committee and articulate any financial conflict of interest relative to the items and discuss why it should be added. The technology assessment committee will take the application and research to an outside third party to review whether the third party believes the claims would be helpful. The physician committee will then determine whether to approve or deny the application. Since instituting this process in 2003, Norton has approved approximately 83% of the applications submitted.

Although new technology is expensive, it is a primary safety issue relative to achieving better patient outcomes. Further, technology has helped Norton avoid spending needlessly by not buying technology that did not meet their overall standards. In an interview George Y. Hersch, system vice president, material management at Norton Healthcare, told us "The cost factor, let's face it ... new technologies add to new cost and rarely is the new technology brought in at a lower cost. Sometimes it's [cost] neutral, but often these companies are trying to recoup their investment and so it's a little difficult to negotiate with some of them." Hersch explains that Norton is focused on cost avoidance versus cost savings. He says if providers want to bring in new technologies that are more expensive, but they can't prove that the technologies have a better clinical outcome or that they are better than what is currently being used than those new technologies will be rejected. "This committee is first and foremost a patient safety committee and a cost avoidance committee for expensive technologies that don't hold any promise," Hersch says.

Clearly, if the new equipment or formulary items would not have ultimately achieved their goals and objectives, it would have increased cost for the health system. Although savings is typically debatable, Norton believes they have done a good job of avoiding acquiring devices considered not worth the clinical risk or unproven.

Savings can also be achieved through various group purchasing organizations. Leaders of larger group purchasing organizations understand the importance of the integrated delivery model (IDM) and health system concept. Norton's national group purchasing organization is creating a platform to service the IDM, as well as work with them collectively to help accomplish their goals and objectives. This may be done by multiple hospitals and by multiple IDMs to consider overall outcomes and approval processes.

Norton Healthcare was also one of the first organizations to go public with their performance and quality data in 2005. Their data is currently accessible at *www.nortonhealthcare.com/body.cfm?id=157.* The data and documentation, while impressive, further illustrates the overall focus on the quality of care and safety elements Norton provides for their patients—roughly 600 nationally recognized quality indicators and practices.

Any organization that aspires to develop an integrated delivery model (IDM) and ACO in the future should keenly study these quality data sets in an effort to achieve the same type of system for their own organization. But where does an organization start? It is always easier to measure processes rather than to measure outcomes; however, that is what Norton strives to do. Ben Yandell, vice president, material management, strongly recommends beginning by hiring a data analyst. Although Yandell does not mean to minimize the importance of software, he strongly believes in the need to have an individual or a team directly involved with the data to begin comparing and setting goals and objectives.

For example, in mid-2010, Norton started a clinical effectiveness initiative that is based on diagnosis-related groups. Two of these include lower extremity joint replacement and congestive heart failure. Based on actions taken within the organization, early data suggests a 38% reduction in their 30-day readmission rates for congestive heart failure and a cost reduction in the 5% range. These types of analyses require a significant commitment to process metrics to measure quality outcomes. Ken Wilson, MD, system vice president, clinical effectiveness and quality, stated it best by saying that Norton is "relentlessly focused on being able to measure outcomes." Likewise, Kevin Stone, director of accountable care development with Dartmouth-Hitchcock, states that they have developed care guidelines attached to various chronic disease conditions. This has allowed them to better understand and organize through best practices for such treatments as hypertension, chronic obstructive pulmonary disease, congestive heart failure, coronary artery disease, and diabetes. They then try to compare to general population statistics to understand better where they have gaps in care. From a preventive care perspective, an example is data showing that a 53-year-old female has not had a mammogram; the patient can be contacted proactively to schedule the exam.

Further, Dartmouth-Hitchcock developed resources to support managing the hospital stay, preventing hospital readmissions, better emergency room use, and various patient cohorts. This has included development of specific post-acute care discharge services to better engage the patient at home to result in better treatment outcomes.

ACOs and various IDMs in the future will be required to achieve such objectives and capabilities. CMS has compared hospital data for years and, similarly, will soon begin comparing physician reports.

Why have organizations like Norton and Dartmouth-Hitchcock been so successful? In an interview for this book, Kevin Stone of Dartmouth-Hitchcock told us, "Our trustees had set as part of our mission population health management and improving the value equation, so we were committed as an organization independent of the Medicare Demonstration program. Trying to deliver care in a way that maximizes the value for a defined population, including developing necessary infrastructure, was work we were committed to doing anyway." Stone says that the Medicare Demonstration program definitely helped sharpen its direction on that path. "While we wouldn't have changed much of what tried to do because of the Demonstration project, our participation really helped us organize and accelerate achieving our aim," he says.

Dartmouth-Hitchcock's trustees set their mission of population health management and improving the value equation early on and committed the organization independent of the Medicare pilot program. They were trying to deliver care in a way that maximized value for a defined population, which drove the infrastructure changes necessary to achieve these objectives. In Stone's opinion, although they were along this path, the Medicare program helped them stay focused on what they were trying to achieve and to accomplish their goals.

The early issues for Dartmouth-Hitchcock were similar to those at Norton Healthcare; they needed to determine how to implement something so significant. For any organization, it will take significant time and investment of resources to get the systems in place.

The necessary investment in infrastructure will include the following action items:

- Getting resources

- Getting organized

- Getting systems in place

- Selecting physicians leaders

The importance of choosing physicians who are natural leaders within the organization cannot be understated. Ideal candidates are physicians who have high clinical credibility, are well respected among their peers, are highly productive, and have specific specialty ties to be able to relate to the other physicians within the organization. With great physician champions that provide strong protocols, the other physicians within the organization should get on board relatively quickly, because most physicians want to improve quality at a lower cost. For Dartmouth-Hitchcock, this included evolving their primary care delivery practices into medical homes in order to qualify as a National Committee for Quality Assurance Level 3 certified medical home. They have focused on 32 quality metrics and chart audits to better assess outcomes. According to Kevin Stone, "The 32 quality metrics were set by Medicare; some were claims-based and some were chart-based. A composite quality score was created from performance ... for each PGP participant." The metrics are available at the CMS website at *www.cms.gov/Quality ImprovementOrgs/downloads/QIO_Improvement_RTC_fnl.pdf.* Dartmouth-Hitchcock generally scored in the 94%–98% range, which has contributed to the success of their overall initiative. (*Note:* Chapter 12 addresses the medical homes concept.) Dartmouth-Hitchcock makes publically available an array of quality metrics that can be accessed at *www.dhmc.org/webpage.cfm?site_id=2&org_id= 459&gsec_id=0&sec_id=0&item_id=20534.*

Over the past five years, the most recent five-year projection period, with approximately 30,000 Medicare members, Dartmouth-Hitchcock's ACO has exceeded its targeted savings by around $35 million. This is important because it increased the quality of care provided and achieved significant savings. The targeted goals were set by the federal government, with a base cost risk adjustment factor compared to their peer group within the market. The government took the first amount of savings achieved through this established Medicare formula, and then the organization shared with them the allowed savings contribution. The shared savings distribution helped Dartmouth recoup some of their investment to initially develop/create their medical homes, generate the case registries, and form the necessary infrastructure for the ACO initiative.

A look at the Norton quality report on their website or Dartmouth-Hitchcock's 32 quality metric comparison data sets demonstrates the need for a significant commitment to information systems within these organizations. Norton estimates that their recently approved technology assessment committee's decision to implement the Epic Corporation's integrated software system over the next 24 months is a major initiative for the organization. (**Note:** Epic makes software for mid- and large-sized medical groups, hospitals, and integrated healthcare organizations— working with customers that include community hospitals, academic facilities, children's organizations, safety net providers, and multihospital systems. Epic's integrated software spans clinical, access, and revenue functions and extends into the home. See Epic's website at *www.epic.com/about-index.php.*) Dartmouth-Hitchcock estimates that it will invest approximately $60 million in information technology structure to effectively manage population health, which is what the ACO is all about. Norton has recently partnered with Microsoft around an intelligent data warehouse product called Amalga. (**Note:** Microsoft® Amalga brings historically disparate data together and makes it easy to identify and act on insights into clinical, financial, or operational performance. Amalga central-izes digital information of all types into a single, continually updated repository that is available for analysis and data sharing. See the Microsoft Amalga website at *www.microsoft.com/en-us/microsofthealth/products/microsoft-amalga.aspx*.) Amalga will allow Norton to combine data from all information systems and then create information reports from the data. This will include hot queries and report writing, which will help them focus on true population health management.

As better quality and outcomes data become available, physician and provider compensation will be affected. Although systems across the country may use typical Physician Quality Reporting System indicators to help supplement current productivity-based models, it is apparent that key matters, such as readmission rates and other outcomes data, will increase as important components for physician compensation. (See Chapter 5 for more information on physician compensation models.)

Healthcare systems will face many challenges in the development of ACOs. Without outside funding or investment, it will be necessary to use or redeploy resources already available. The success of the Norton Healthcare and Dartmouth-Hitchcock programs is due to the continued focused efforts on achieving their established goals, their commitment to quality and outcomes, and their invest-ment in infrastructure through technology solutions and leadership teams.

Many organizations may tend to believe in their past successes and feel as if they have everything under control. The one consistent theme throughout the interviews conducted for this chapter, outside of the overall goals and objectives, is the need to continue the relentless pursuit to evolve their organizations; otherwise, they anticipate setbacks in performance. Every organization must have everyone on the same page; that is, everyone must understand the work that is required and the commitment that must be made to be successful.

Author's note: The discussion of products and companies in this chapter does not constitute a recommendation by the author. The identification of products is in the context of reporting from Norton Healthcare and Dartmouth-Hitchcock.

Glossary of Acronyms

ACO	Accountable Care Organization
ASC	Ambulatory surgery center
ASP	Application service provider
BY	Benchmark year
CHR	Community health records
CMS	Centers for Medicare & Medicaid Services
CNS	Clinical nurse specialist
CPOE	Computerized physician order entry
DOJ	Department of Justice
DRG	Diagnosis-related groups
ED	Emergency department
EHR	Electronic health records
EMTALA	Emergency Medical Treatment and Active Labor Act
ESRD	End-stage renal disease
FFS	Fee-for-service
FQHC	Federally qualified health center
FTC	Federal Trade Commission
GPRO	Group Practice Reporting Option

HCC	Hierarchical Condition Category
HCPCS	Healthcare Common Procedure Coding System
HHS	Department of Health and Human Services
HIE	Health information exchange
HIT	Health information technology
HMO	Health maintenance organization
IDM	Integrated delivery model
IPA	Independent Practice Association
IRS	Internal Revenue Service
ISO	Information services organization
IT	Information technology
LIS	Laboratory information systems
M&A	Mergers and acquisitions
MA	Medicare Advantage
MedPAC	Medicare Payment Advisory Commission
MPI	Master patient index
MSO	Management services organization
MSR	Minimum savings rate
NCQA	National Committee for Quality Assurance
NP	Nurse practitioner
NPI	National provider identifier
NQF	National Quality Forum
OIG	Office of Inspector General
PA	Physician assistance
PACS	Picture archiving and communication system
PCMH	Patient-centered medical home

PCP	Primary care physician
PHO	Physician-hospital organization
POS	Point of service
PPACA	Patient Protection and Affordable Care Act
PPM	Physician practice management
PPO	Preferred provider organization
PPS	Prospective payment system
PQRI	Physician Quality Reporting Initiative (now called PQRS)
PQRS	Physician Quality Reporting System
PSA	Professional Services Agreement and Primary Service Area (unrelated)
RBRVS	Resource-based relative value scale
RHC	Rural health clinic
RHIO	Regional health information organizations
RIS	Radiology information systems
SaaS	Software as a service
SSP	Shared Savings Program
TIN	Tax identification number
WHO	World Health Organization
wRVU	Work relative value unit